"In this riveting memoir, journalist Tessa Miller describes tne sudden onset of severe Crohn's disease in her twenties. . . . Evocative . . . She analyzes studies and statistics about health care and chronic illness in the U.S., including racial and gender discrimination. It's a fascinating and disturbing read."

—*BuzzFeed*

"[Miller] writes with precision, conviction, respect, and thoughtfulness about pain as well as the disparate, and at times unjust, experiences that people face when navigating the American healthcare system. . . . *What Doesn't Kill You* is relentlessly researched and undeniably smart, but more than that, it is humane and offers reliable information to chronically ill people and their allies."

—*The New York Times*

"[Miller] puts her experiences to paper, detailing the many ways her life changed after her diagnosis . . . all in a digestible, authentic manner. . . . As applicable and important a read as ever."

—*Shape*

"More than a memoir . . . [Miller] offers hard-earned wisdom, solidarity, and hope for others facing the medical, occupational, and social realities inherent in receiving a lifetime diagnosis."

—*Life & Style*

"Miller weaves together her harrowing story of navigating the health-care system with frank and funny observations about living with an invisible disease, making this a must-read."

—*OK!* (UK)

"Powerful and moving . . . A source of hope and comfort for those living with a long-term ailment."   —*Star*

"Chronically ill people, their loved ones, and their colleagues will find useful advice and food for thought in this conversational, revealing memoir and guide. . . . [A] page-turner and a quality resource."   —*Booklist*

"A clear, no-holds-barred account that will be useful both to those coming to grips with their own chronic illness and to the people in their lives."   —*Library Journal*

"*What Doesn't Kill You* would have been engrossing as a memoir of illness and infuriating as a polemic against the dysfunctional, often malicious American health-care system. Instead, through skill and deep insight, it manages to be even more. Equal parts personal history, polemic, and guidebook, its service journalism is invaluable for those living with 'a body in revolt,' as Miller puts it. The dividing line between the land of the well and that of the sick is an often blurry one, and Miller documents life on its uncertain borders with clarity and force."

—Anna Merlan, author of *Republic of Lies*

"This is a must-read book for anyone suffering from chronic illness and for the people who care for them. Beautifully written and full of keen personal observations, *What Doesn't Kill You* is a powerful memoir and a smart self-help book rolled into one. Living with an invisible disability like Crohn's is a lonely business, but Tessa Miller makes you feel less alone. Her voice is funny, helpful, and most of all honest—she doesn't sugarcoat the truth, which is that life with a chronic disease is really damn

hard. But you don't have to be hard on yourself, too. There are ways to ease the pain, both mental and physical, and this book is a good place to start learning what that means."
—Annalee Newitz, bestselling author of *Autonomous* and *Scatter, Adapt, and Remember*

"A book you don't just read but inhabit. Tessa Miller powerfully captures all the pain and beauty of being alive in this beautiful hybrid of memoir and journalism. If you have a chronic illness, *What Doesn't Kill You* will make you feel seen; to everyone else, it offers the opportunity to listen without judgment and, ultimately, to care about bodies different from your own."
—Samantha Allen, author of *Real Queer America*

"Unflinchingly honest, *What Doesn't Kill You* provides an unfiltered look at what it truly means to be sick. Miller takes her years navigating the health-care system and distills them into crucial resources and eye-opening insights. A must-read for those trying to navigate life with a chronic illness."
—Jordan Davidson, cofounder of Endo Warriors and women's health advocate

"Breathtaking. Miller brings together an absolutely frank personal memoir with scientific accuracy about her disease and insights into relationships, the mind-body connection, and our broken health system. She turns her life into an affirming guidebook to living with warmth, compassion, humor, humility, and generosity. This book will make you want to be a better friend, colleague, daughter, son, sibling, and partner."
—Esther Choo, MD, MPH, associate professor of emergency medicine and cofounder of Equity Quotient

"This is a book to press into someone's hands and say, 'Read this.' It both makes you feel you really know the author and makes you want to spend more time with her to get to know her better. *What Doesn't Kill You* is by turns harrowing, heartbreaking, funny, and practical, but it is compassionate on every single page. It is a book for people with chronic illness, people who love someone with a chronic illness, people who care for patients with chronic illnesses, and people who may one day develop a chronic illness. In other words, it is a book for everyone."

—Daniel Summers, MD, *Slate* and *Daily Beast* columnist

WHAT DOESN'T KILL YOU

A LIFE WITH CHRONIC ILLNESS—
LESSONS FROM A BODY IN REVOLT

TESSA MILLER

A HOLT PAPERBACK
HENRY HOLT AND COMPANY
NEW YORK

Holt Paperbacks
Henry Holt and Company
Publishers since 1866
120 Broadway
New York, New York 10271
www.henryholt.com

A Holt Paperback® and ⓗ® are registered trademarks of Macmillan Publishing Group, LLC.

The Library of Congress has cataloged the hardcover edition as follows:

Names: Miller, Tessa, 1988– author.
Title: What doesn't kill you : a life with chronic illness—lessons from a
body in revolt / Tessa Miller.
Description: First edition. | New York : Henry Holt and Company, 2021. |
Includes bibliographical references and index.
Identifiers: LCCN 2020035130 (print) | LCCN 2020035131 (ebook) | ISBN
9781250751454 (hardcover) | ISBN 9781250751461 (ebook)
Subjects: LCSH: Miller, Tessa, 1988—Health | Crohn's
disease—Patients—New York (State)—New York—Biography.
Classification: LCC RC862.E52 M55 2021 (print) | LCC RC862.E52 (ebook) |
DDC 616.3/440092 [B]—dc23
LC record available at https://lccn.loc.gov/2020035130
LC ebook record available at https://lccn.loc.gov/2020035131

ISBN: 9781250751478 (trade paperback)

Our books may be purchased in bulk for promotional, educational, or business use. Please
contact your local bookseller or the Macmillan Corporate and Premium Sales Department at
(800) 221-7945, extension 5442, or by email at MacmillanSpecialMarkets@macmillan.com.

Originally published in hardcover in 2021 by Henry Holt and Company

First Holt Paperbacks Edition 2022

Designed by Steven Seighman

Printed in the United States of America

D   10   9   8   7   6   5   4   3

For Zoe

Be kind to me, or treat me mean
I'll make the most of it,
I'm an extraordinary machine

—FIONA APPLE

Contents

Author's Note

This is a book of nonfiction. It's part memoir, detailing the story of my illness—Crohn's disease—and all its spindly legs, how it stretches forward and back through the timeline of my years, and how it shook up my body and my brain in ways I wasn't ready for. I've written the autobiographical part of this book through memories, journals, old social media posts, medical records, and interviews with my family and my doctors. Parts of this book have appeared in various forms in the *New York Times*, the *Daily Beast*, *Medium*, and *Self*. My writing here deals with details of bowel disease, as well as hospitalization, sexual assault, and physical and emotional abuse. Certain names and identifying details have been changed or omitted.

This book is also part guide for fellow chronically ill people—meaning those with incurable conditions—and their loved ones, sharing the lessons I've learned from my diagnosis through today. This is the book I wish someone had given me, as well as the book I wish someone had given my family and friends, when I got sick. I didn't need conflicting texts about what I should or shouldn't eat or dry clinical reports or self-help books written by able-bodied authors offering little more than "reduce stress."

I needed a book written by someone who exists in that foggy space between the common cold and terminal cancer, where illness doesn't go away but won't kill you. I needed someone who lives *every single day* with illness to tell me that 1) I wasn't alone and 2) my life was going to change in unexpected, difficult, and surprisingly beautiful ways.

This isn't a book about what causes chronic illness or what might cure it. I do not speculate about treatment for others, I only describe my own. With help from people far smarter than I am, I tell readers both what I wish I knew before I got sick forever and what I know now, a decade later: how to find doctors who won't dismiss your symptoms, how to navigate changing relationships and careers, how to grieve a self that doesn't exist anymore, why mental health care is so important, and how joy is possible despite (and because of) it all. If you're interested in my personal story, that's generally at the beginning of each chapter, followed by the more service journalism–based writing. But the book also has appendices and an index, so you can search for particular topics that matter to you. Choose your own adventure.

I picked the mental health experts interviewed in this book for their areas of specialization as well as their varied approaches; you'll notice that almost all have backgrounds in health psychology or concentrate in the overlap of chronic illness and mental health. Some practice cognitive behavioral therapy while others focus on psychoanalysis; some are nondiagnostic while others work within diagnostic parameters; some work with individuals while others specialize in couples or families. I thank them deeply for offering their time and expertise on the phone and through email, and I thank my mom for her hours transcribing these interviews.

For me, chronic illness and its psychological, social, and economic aftershocks brought with it an intense need to be understood. I imagine anyone who writes a memoir has that need as well. I hope that if you're chronically ill and you read this book, you will feel seen. If you've dealt with trauma of mind, body, or both, I hope you will read this book and feel less alone. And if you're not chronically ill or if you love someone who is, I hope you will read this book and understand all of us better.

A quick note on the language in this book: *Chronically ill* technically means any illness lasting longer than three months, but the discussion in this book means illness that does not go away—it can be managed but not cured. Chronic illness does not usually cause death (though complications of chronic illness can and do kill). *Terminal illness*, on the other hand, cannot be cured and ends in death. Some illnesses, like HIV, that were once terminal are now considered chronic because good treatment exists. *Disability* includes any mental, physical, intellectual, or sensory impairment. Sometimes, chronic illness and disability overlap; sometimes, chronic illness leads to disability and vice versa. Some people identify as chronically ill but not disabled, disabled but not chronically ill, or chronically ill and disabled. *Able-bodied* means not disabled. (Some people also use *non-disabled*.) I use "chronically ill people" and "disabled people" rather than "people with chronic illness" or "people with disabilities" because this is the language my community prefers.

CHAPTER 1

Blood

The first time I heard of Crohn's disease, I was in fourth grade. 1997. Mom and my fourteen-year-old sister, Kaetlyn, were talking in the front seats of our Ford Escort after school; I was eavesdropping in the back. A girl in Kaetlyn's class was sick with something called Crohn's disease—"that poor thing," Mom kept repeating, barely above a whisper.

"What's Crow's disease?" I asked.

Kaetlyn craned her neck around, slowly and dramatically, eyes in a permanent teenage roll. *"Crohn's* disease," she said, circling her lips around the O, "is where you poop . . . until you *die.*"

I didn't ask any more questions. It was the one of the worst things I'd ever heard.

Fifteen years later, I listened, upright in a hospital bed, as doctors diagnosed me with it.

It was 2012, my second year in New York City. I'd moved to New York in October 2010 from the Midwest for a three-month-long internship at Condé Nast, the storied publisher of *Vogue* and *Vanity Fair* and the *New Yorker*. At the three-month mark, the Condé Nast magazine *Wired* hired me full-time, so what was supposed to be ninety short days turned into ten years (and counting). I've lived in New York City longer, now, than in any other place. I chose it for the same reasons everyone else does: because it's big and weird and everyone here is smarter and weirder than me. Everyone who moves to New York from someplace you've never heard of has got something to prove: that we're intelligent, that we're creative, that we made it out of our hometowns. When I finished four years at Northwestern, the people I graduated with all had a plan: Google or an ad agency or a newspaper. They each seemed to have an uncle who could get them a job. I had no plan, no prospects, no connections. I moved in with Mom and my stepdad in rural Illinois and wore pajamas all day while I watched *House Hunters*, scrolled job listings, and counted down my student loan grace period.

One late summer afternoon just after my twenty-second birthday, I came across what seemed like a fake ad on Craigslist for a public relations internship at Condé Nast (why would one of the world's largest publishers use Craigslist?), specifically working for Chris Anderson's *Wired* as well as a sparse little website called Reddit that, for reasons no one really understood, was doing bonkers traffic. They invited me to an in-person interview, and though PR hadn't crossed my mind as a career option, I knew it meant working closely with writers and editors. In New York, I stayed with a friend from college whose family rented a two-story penthouse above the now-closed Topshop on Broadway. I'd only ever seen homes like it in movies, but my friend and her family moved about it like it belonged to them. Rich people have a way of moving around the world like that, with ownership. I borrowed a black polyester pencil skirt from Kaetlyn and slicked my hair into a bun because that seemed elegant.

In the cab to 4 Times Square, I prayed the internship listing wasn't a con. At the end of a forty-five-minute interview, two intimidating and chic twentysomethings offered me the internship but with a condition: Condé Nast required its interns to be enrolled in college so that the company could give school credit instead of any payment beyond a $12/day—that's $240/month—"travel stipend." I had just graduated, so I would have to reenroll. I used $1,400—most of what I'd saved from my college receptionist job—to buy ¼ credit at Northwestern, enough to make me legit for the company's requirements. Mom and my stepdad agreed to help with three months of rent in hopes that the internship would lead to a real job. I was desperate to get to New York because it felt like everyone else my age was building their lives and I'd be damned if I stayed behind any longer in my pajamas. Even $12 a day felt like progress because that $12 was in New York Freakin' City.

When I moved from Illinois to New York that October, I traveled with just two bags: a tote stitched with my initials, gifted from Mom who monograms everything, and a black suitcase that I bought for $30 at Walmart. Those bags carried everything I needed—and everything I had, really—to fill my shared apartment, a converted one-bedroom on Ludlow and Delancey on the Lower East Side. I found it, too, on Craigslist, and had corresponded via email for several weeks with my soon-to-be roommate, a fellow Midwesterner and recent college grad who would later become a close friend. My room was seven feet by nine feet and pre-painted bright, almost neon orangey red, with a makeshift plywood platform that I put a squeaky Kmart air mattress on. The shower was in the kitchen next to the sink and shared its plumbing, so the tub drain clogged with bits of macaroni noodles and coffee grounds and whatever else got rinsed down the sink. Sometimes during a shower, I'd find myself standing in ankle-deep swamp water. The toilet was in its own closet with a narrow window that overlooked the backyard of the next-door karaoke bar, where you could listen to drunk people singing along to Whitney Houston and Bon Jovi while you peed, whether you wanted to or not. A vegetable warehouse was downstairs, and the smell of rotting onions wafted down the block most days. Our middle-aged neighbor smoked cigarettes in the hallway while wearing tighty-whities and a hot pink wig. Garbage piled so high in the first-floor hallway, where the trash cans lived, that those tenants' front doors got blocked in. Cockroaches scattered when you turned on our kitchen light. The room cost $750/month and I loved it well for more than a year, until bed bugs forced me to flee to Brooklyn.

If I was from Earth, Condé Nast was Mars. Even my four years at Northwestern, moving among the children of senators and diplomats and CEOs, hadn't prepared me for the world of prestige publishing. A boss's boss told me I was "too nice" to succeed. A creative director grabbed my ass at a company retreat. Friends in ad sales passed along tales of cocaine-fueled parties and affairs between C-titles and their assistants. My colleagues used words like *summer* as a verb and bonded over which posh camp they'd gone to as adolescents. In my hometown, no one went to camp—we detasseled corn, babysat, and hung out at whoever's house had the aboveground pool. And at Condé Nast, people cared a lot about appearance. Though I stayed mostly outside of that bubble working for tech publications, I couldn't help but interact with the fashion set (even Ms. Wintour herself) in the lobby and the cafeteria. I watched them as though we were separated by glass, knowing that we would never be alike—though whiteness and thinness and a maxed-out thousand-dollar-limit credit card I used for clothing allowed me to pass unnoticed. My two years at Condé Nast were less about learning how to write press releases or monitor media impressions and more of an education in the ways of a ruling class.

In early 2012, I jumped at the opportunity for an editorship at the famous how-to site Lifehacker. By then, I lived in a boxy two-bedroom in South Williamsburg, right where hipsters and Hasids start to overlap. I was soon making $49,000 a year plus small monetary bonuses for pageviews, and I felt like I was *rolling in it*. I wanted to upgrade luggage for my Thanksgiving trip back to Illinois, so I walked less than a mile from my apartment to a row of family-run shops where the Satmar store owner helped me choose a practical rolling suitcase. As I handed over my debit card to pay for the bag, searing cramps gripped my abdomen. I grabbed the receipt, rushed out of the store, and wheeled my way home. The pain made it so hard to breathe that I doubled over at crosswalks. "Don't shit yourself, please don't shit yourself, *don't you dare* shit yourself," I said under my breath. By sheer will and Herculean clenching, I didn't. But I spent the rest of the night going from my bed to the toilet—bed to toilet—bed to toilet—while my intestines tortured me.

I'd experienced stomach pain all my life but this was something else. My guts were being pulled like taffy and shredded with hot razor blades. The cramping felt as though a man with large fists had reached inside my body and was wringing my colon like a damp rag. The next morning, my mouth and throat exploded with throbbing lumps, akin to canker sores on steroids. I swallowed a handful of Tylenol and Imodium and caught my flight to Illinois, sweaty and white-knuckled the whole way.

Instead of getting better at Mom's house, I declined further. My family celebrated Thanksgiving while I stayed upstairs, leaving bed only to go to the bathroom ten, twenty, thirty times a day—filling the toilet bowl with nothing but bright red blood and bits of intestinal tissue that floated like scritta paper. Seeing blood for the first time from my body, outside of my body, when it wasn't supposed to be there, was distressing and scary—but more than that, it felt like a total loss of control. I didn't know the source and I couldn't stop it. Every time I went to the bathroom, there was more red. Meanwhile, the pain escalated. It felt like I was shitting barbed wire. I didn't want to eat—even a drink of water had me running to the toilet within seconds. Mouth sores continued to spread and scatter down my tongue and across my tonsils, making it excruciating to speak or swallow. I started soiling myself trying to walk the fifteen steps from the bedroom to the bathroom.

I'd had stomach problems for as long as I could remember, but never with bleeding. As Mom tells it, I cried relentlessly until my first birthday; if I wasn't sleeping, I was crying. Some nights the only way I'd sleep was chest-to-chest with Dad, who used my diapered butt as a book prop so he could keep up with his PhD reading. A pediatrician ruled it colic and said I'd grow out of it. In second grade, I had stomachaches so severe that I'd double over at school. My teacher sent me to the guidance counselor, who asked if I was crying for attention. In fifth grade, I had a bout of illness—abdominal pain and vomiting—that kept me out of school for a month. A CT scan at the local children's hospital was inconclusive. Freshman year of college, another monthlong illness with ER visits and no certain diagnosis. Fear, stress, or excitement led to cramping pain and diarrhea, so early on, I was labeled "sensitive" and a "nervous kid." Mom used to ask if I just had butterflies in my stomach and I'd say, "Not butterflies. Killer bees." Any excessive collegiate drinking made me not just hungover, but sick for days. My peers got headaches and bounced back with a greasy cheeseburger, but I'd be vomiting and pooping for at least forty-eight hours. During my first year in New York, I'd sometimes get gripping stomach pain accompanied by a sore rash on my hands and face.

I got used to it all.

But blood was different. Blood meant something was really wrong. I'd planned for everything else, but I had never thought to plan for blood. I signed up for every high school extracurricular, graduated at the top of my class, stayed out of trouble (for the most part), made it out of my little farm town, did four years at Northwestern, moved to New York, secured a full-time job with a 401(k), and paid my student loans on time. I was going to work my way up the media ladder and become the editor in chief of something by the time I turned thirty, *goddammit*. But now, I was bleeding uncontrollably from my butthole.

No.

No.

NO.

"I need to go to the emergency room," I told Mom.

My folks' rural Illinois community, where they settled after their marriage in 2006, is one hundred miles south of Chicago and thirty miles north of where I went to high school. Thousands of years ago this part of Illinois was quite rugged, but glaciers leveled it into miles of land fit for crops and interstate, gridded and flat like a board game. Now it's car country. Flyover country. Their town has about twelve thousand people and one Catholic hospital out by the interstate. Most residents work there, at the maximum-security prison, or at the manufacturing plant where my stepdad spent forty years. The town has a beautiful 1870s courthouse and pristine square next to dozens of empty storefronts. Opiates are in high demand, and the public schools are suffering from mismanagement and budget cuts. Most businesses have had to install video gambling to stay afloat. But despite the town's problems, people there are friendly, quick to ask how you're doing or lend you a snowblower or bring you a casserole. (Don't be fooled, though: Generations of repressed rage live just below midwestern nice.)

I had been to the ER there once before, the time I was sick freshman year during winter break. The emergency department was not at all like the vast expanses in New York with rows and rows of curtained-off beds and hundreds of people shuffling about. It had ten beds and the same number of seats in the waiting area. One doctor and a handful of nurses. Like the last time I visited, a nurse took me back right away when I told her my symptoms and the doctor saw me quickly. He was in his early thirties, with floppy brown hair and dark-rimmed glasses, and seemed nice enough. He scanned what the nurse had jotted in my chart.

"Bleeding during bowel movements?"

"Yes, rectal bleeding. I'm filling the toilet bowl to the brim with blood."

"And you're sure it isn't menstrual bleeding?"

"Yes, I'm sure."

"Some women have very heavy periods, you know."

He insisted on giving me a rectal exam that I was not ready for nor did I want. I didn't know yet how to advocate for myself. Instead, I cried. That was the beginning of relinquishing my body to health-care professionals, a dehumanization that I'm used to now but will never be okay with. After an hour and a few more tests, the doctor told me he wasn't sure what was wrong, but he suspected some sort of infection. He sent me home with broad-spectrum antibiotics that did nothing for my symptoms except add vomiting.

The toilet kept filling with what looked like pulpy red juice, and the pain remained unbearable. I'd lost all control of my bowels, so I'd just lie on the bathroom floor, pressing my face into the cold tile. My parents eventually stepped in, taking me back to the same ER where the are-you-sure-it's-not-your-period doctor said I was beyond his capacity. An ambulance shuttled me to a bigger Catholic hospital forty miles away, where I spent several days getting poked and prodded and scoped but didn't mind so much thanks to the warm intravenous painkillers. When it was time to drink a gallon of laxative colonoscopy prep, I got halfway through and couldn't stand to swallow any more. "Keep going!" the nurse chirped each time she checked on me. "You can do it!" I couldn't do it. Mom snuck the other half into my hospital room's bathroom and poured it down the sink.

I didn't know then that my life had changed forever. That I'd be able to divide my experiences into before I got sick and after I got sick. The following weeks, months, and years brought short and long hospital stays, good and bad doctors, countless medications: antibiotics, steroids, anti-inflammatories, blood thinners, enemas, rectal foams, antispasmodics, antiemetics, opiates, suppositories, laxatives, biologics, blood plasma, potassium chloride, medicated mouthwash, antidepressants, sleeping pills, probiotics, benzodiazepines, weight-gain supplements, and antivirals; many side effects: hair loss, joint pain, migraines, hives, throat swelling, mood swings, appetite changes, intestinal blockages, bowel impactions, insomnia, and fatigue; multiple diagnoses, blood tests, stool tests, CT scans, X-rays, colonoscopies, giant hospital bills and fights with insurance companies, and three fecal microbiota transplants (yes, that means someone else's stool transferred to my digestive tract).

I became a professional patient, and a good one. I learned that bodies can be inexplicably resilient and curiously fragile. I would never get better, and that would change *everything*: the way I think about my body, my health, my relationships, my work, and my life. When things get rough, people like to say, "this too shall pass." But what happens when "this" never goes away?

As I got to know hundreds of chronically ill folks over the coming years through my work as a journalist and via my support groups, it became clear that chronic illness's physical symptoms are one small part of an intricate puzzle. We're heroic when it comes to pain—it's the mental Olympics that challenge us: the depression and anxiety that come along with a malfunctioning body; the defeat of visiting doctor after doctor only to hear it's "all in your head"; the sick, sleepless nights worried about health insurance; the hope of a new treatment and the crushing loss when it doesn't work; the longing for loved ones to understand that you're the same you—*except not*; the grieving of a self that doesn't exist anymore; the PTSD from long hospital stays and invasive procedures; the new rules of an unrecognizable body; the inescapable loneliness. Most conversation about chronic illness—and there isn't much of it, publicly—focuses on the physical. But forever sickness, I would learn, changes more than bones and blood. It changes goals, careers, intimate relationships, families, and dreams.

At the hospital, a colonoscopy, biopsies, X-rays, and a CT scan confirmed the diagnosis of inflammatory bowel disease (IBD). All five sections of my colon—sigmoid, descending, transverse, ascending, and cecum—and my rectum were riddled with inflammation and ulceration. IBD (not to be confused with irritable bowel syndrome, IBS) is a chronic disease that causes the immune system to attack the digestive system. There are two kinds of IBD: Crohn's disease, which affects the entire digestive system from mouth to anus, and ulcerative colitis (UC), which is contained to the large intestine (also called the colon). Crohn's and UC can range from mild to severe and will often progress if not treated. Both are notoriously difficult to diagnose, as the symptoms can point to other illnesses, and it isn't uncommon for it to take a long time to get a proper diagnosis. As I wrote in a piece for the *New York Times*, IBD results in what has always seemed to me to be the attempted birth of my intestines through my butthole. Like many chronic diseases, IBD works in patterns of flares and remissions; no one is quite sure what causes either, though there are several theories, and how long each flare or remission lasts varies wildly from patient to patient. I've tried to describe IBD in a way people without the disease might understand: Think of the worst food poisoning or norovirus you've ever had, then times it by one hundred, for the rest of your life. But even that doesn't come close to capturing the pain. You can't know it until you're there.

An estimated three million people and rising in the United States have IBD,[1] and most of us are diagnosed before the age of thirty-five. Though autoimmune diseases are much more common in women than men (in the United States, 80 percent of the country's 23.5 million autoimmune disease patients are women[2]), men and women are at about the same risk for IBD.[3] IBD patients try medication after medication—including aminosalicylates, corticosteroids, immunomodulators, antibiotics, and biologics—attempting to manage the disease and, hopefully, reach remission. (Some new research suggests that patients who don't respond to medication might benefit from stem cell therapy, which is still in the clinical trial phase.[4]) Many IBD patients, including 70 percent of Crohn's patients,[5] go on to have surgical intervention that might include having parts of their bowels removed or resectioned. Some live with temporary or permanent ostomies—external pouches that collect waste from rerouted intestines; or J-pouches—internal pouches formed by removing the colon and rectum and connecting the small intestine to the anus.

1. Data and Statistics: "Inflammatory Bowel Disease Prevalence (IBD) in the United States," Centers for Disease Control and Prevention; accessed February 3, 2020, https://www.cdc.gov/ibd/data-statistics.htm.

2. "Autoimmune Disease: Why Is My Immune System Attacking Itself?," Johns Hopkins Medicine; accessed February 3, 2020, https://www.hopkinsmedicine.org/health/wellness-and-prevention/autoimmune-disease-why-is-my-immune-system-attacking-itself.

3. "The Facts About Inflammatory Bowel Diseases," Crohn's and Colitis Foundation, updated 2014.

4. Hiromichi Shimizu et al., "Stem Cell–Based Therapy for Inflammatory Bowel Disease," *Intestinal Research* 17, no. 3 (2019): 311–16.

5. "Crohn's Disease Treatment Options," Crohn's and Colitis Foundation; accessed February 2, 2020, https://www.crohnscolitisfoundation.org/What-is-crohns-disease/treatment.

Now here's where I list all the scary, painful stuff IBD can cause, like ulceration and bleeding throughout the digestive tract, diarrhea, vomiting, dehydration, malnutrition (IBD guts have a hard time absorbing nutrients), fatigue, fistulas (abnormal connections between organs; rectovaginal fistulas are a common topic of conversation in my support groups), bowel perforations (holes in the intestines), scar tissue in the digestive tract, fissures (tears in tissue that often cause bleeding), abscesses, joint pain and arthritis, anemia, eye inflammation and vision problems, and tooth decay. During childhood, IBD can cause stunted growth and delayed puberty.[6] It can also trigger something called toxic megacolon, which sounds like a death metal band but is in reality a life-threatening expansion and distension of the colon that traps gas and stool to the point of rupture. (You know the chest-burster scene in *Alien*? That was written by a guy with Crohn's. He died from complications of the disease.) IBD also increases the risk of digestive cancers, and people with IBD are more likely to struggle with other chronic illnesses including cardiovascular disease, respiratory disease, kidney and liver disease, and arthritis. (Many chronically ill folks have more than one illness, as they often come in twos and threes and sometimes more. Multiple diagnoses are not at all strange in the chronic illness community. Think of it like any structure: If one part begins to crumble, others are likely to follow.) On top of these symptoms, the drugs that treat IBD trigger significant side effects, like hair loss, joint pain, drug-induced lupus, and even cancer.

6. Phyllis Brown, "Boys Three Times More Likely to Have Growth Delay with Crohn's," University of California San Francisco, last updated December 4, 2007; accessed March 3, 2020, https://www.ucsf.edu/news/2007/12/5646/boys -three-times-more-likely-have-growth-delay-crohns.

It's an unfair, heartless, and often debilitating disease.

Each patient is unique—chronically ill people, even with the same diagnosis, aren't a monolith. My flare-ups tend to happen like this: First, I start to experience pain and gas. Not regular gas, like everyone gets—painful gas that bloats my belly so badly that I look several months pregnant. Inflammation and ulceration, combined with scar tissue from previous flares, make it difficult for gas to move its way out of my body, so it becomes trapped and extremely uncomfortable. Next comes the blood—initially, just a little on the toilet paper. Then more. Then a lot, often with clotting. As it increases, so does my sense of dread. Mucus mixes with the blood along with intestinal tissue, and at a certain point I stop passing stool and start passing only that bloody mixture. As the flare progresses, I cannot control my bowels at all. I have accidents. I get sores in my mouth and throat that must be treated with a numbing rinse called "magic mouthwash" that was created for the oral burns experienced during cancer treatment. The 1-to-10 pain scale is highly subjective, but my flare pain hovers around a 7 with some higher bursts; when it gets above that, I go to the ER because it becomes unmanageable without IV opioids and doctor intervention. But I'm at high risk for hospital-acquired infections, so even going to the ER comes with major hazards. It's frightening that the place I'm supposed to go to get better can make me even sicker.

During flares, I get a painful, swollen sensation that feels like someone is playing an off-rhythm drum in my rectum at all hours, day and night. My rectum fills with fluid that makes it feel like I need to go to the bathroom constantly; this is when passing gas becomes a dangerous game of *Will She Shit Herself?* (insert game show music here). I experience waves of cramps so agonizing that I moan as though I'm laboring. I throw up because of the pain. Because of intestinal narrowing due to new inflammation and old scar tissue, I often get blockages and impactions; blockages occur when the intestine is too narrow for anything to pass through, and impactions happen when stool becomes trapped and immobile. Both cause the sort of pain that makes me leave my body and crawl on the ceiling. The whole point of the digestive system is to get stuff *out*, but impactions and blockages make that impossible. And on already inflamed, scarred-up guts? I don't know the words to describe the misery.

More often than not, I also get swelling and stiffness in my joints, nausea, fatigue, and weakness. During flares, my blood panels show borderline or full-blown anemia, high inflammation markers like exponentially increased white cell counts and off-the-charts C-reactive protein (CRP), and decreased electrolytes. My flares, so far, have lasted weeks or months; some unlucky IBD-ers have yearslong flare-ups with little to no relief. I also get "mini flares" that last a few days at a time but remedy themselves, and my disease always flares up during my period as hormones like estrogen can increase IBD symptoms. I've reached remission twice, and (knock on wood) am currently in the longest remission—almost three years—since my diagnosis. Remission doesn't mean I'm cured or even that I don't have symptoms; it basically means I have no signs of active disease via colonoscopy.

That Thanksgiving, in the Midwest, I was initially diagnosed with UC, the form of IBD contained to the large intestine. Later, when I got more comprehensive medical care, that diagnosis changed to "indeterminate IBD," and then Crohn's disease. (I was also diagnosed with celiac disease, an immune response in the small intestine to gluten, a sticky protein found in wheat, barley, and rye that's managed with a strict gluten-free diet. For the sake of not confusing the reader, I will refer to my disease as Crohn's or IBD.) But that November in Illinois, when I dove into research about my diagnosis, I didn't know what "chronic" meant in any real sense. I started taking four large maroon pills called mesalamine every day and tweaked my diet. I didn't need to go to the bathroom as urgently or frequently, and when I did go, there was less blood. I felt strong enough to fly back to New York, return to my job, and find some semblance of a normal twenty-four-year-old's life.

Wishful thinking.

Two weeks passed and my symptoms came back fiercer than before, along with new, troubling ones. The urgency and blood were there, now with violent, green, mucus-laden diarrhea. Going to the bathroom caused so much pain that I'd simultaneously vomit; a few times I couldn't make it to the toilet, so I shit my pants while forcefully vomiting into whatever plastic bag I could grab in time. My bedroom accumulated tied-off Walgreens bags full of puke that I was too weak to carry to the building's trash can, and I threw away pair after pair of soiled underwear and pajama bottoms.

One morning before dawn, after being sick for hours in the apartment's shared bathroom, as the toilet rapidly overflowed, I realized that I'd clogged it. Green diarrhea, blood, and vomit pooled across the bathroom floor as I panicked and searched for the plunger, which seemed to have disappeared. (Turns out we never had one.) My roommate, a subletter from the internet, was still asleep, and at this point I'd managed to keep my illness secret from her. So I scrambled to the closest drugstore and returned with a plunger, gloves, a bucket, and bleach. On hands and knees, I frantically removed the evidence of my rotting, broken body.

Along with the diarrhea and vomiting came a high fever, stiff joint pain, and a distended abdomen that frightened me to look at. My limbs were so thin but my belly remained swollen. I didn't know whose body I saw in the mirror. Panicked, I asked Mom to come to New York to help look after me. When she saw how much I'd deteriorated since putting me on a plane two weeks earlier, her eyes turned fearful.

"You're coming back to Illinois with me," she said. It wasn't a question—it was a decision. I tried to argue I wasn't *that* sick. That I could handle it. That the doctor said I'd have flare-ups and this was probably one of them. That I didn't look *so* terrible, did I? We screamed at each other until she left in a taxi, on her way to the airport without me. It took me less than five minutes to realize I might die if I stayed.

"Mom, I changed my mind," I cried through the phone. Her cab was waiting outside minutes later.

As quickly as she'd flown in, she was flying back—this time with a sick kid who wouldn't remember anything of that flight. "We wandered the parking lot at O'Hare Airport looking for my car and I knew you were so close to giving up," Mom told me. "That was the first time I thought you might die."

A hundred miles of Interstate 55 later, I was back in the central Illinois hospital I'd been so glad to leave.

A stool test revealed that I had an infection called *Clostridium difficile*, sometimes called *Clostridioides difficile* (as in "difficult"), or *C. diff* for short, a spore-forming bacteria that's extremely contagious and hard to treat. Common in hospitals, nursing homes, and other health-care centers where antibiotic use is high and compromised immune systems are common, *C. diff* releases toxins that attack the lining of the large intestine. It causes aggressive, foul-smelling diarrhea, an increased white blood cell count, dehydration, fever, and abdominal bloating. If it isn't treated properly, *C. diff* can kill you. It infects about 500,000 people every year in the United States and kills 30,000[7]—a historically high number, thanks in part to increasing antibiotic resistance. To put that in perspective, car accidents kill about 32,000.

The doctors swiftly isolated me and started a regimen of vancomycin, an expensive antibiotic ($2,000 per course without insurance) that's a first-line treatment against *C. diff*. It seems counterintuitive that *C. diff* most often happens *because of* antibiotics and is then *treated with* antibiotics, but that's the protocol. Anyone coming into my room, limited to hospital staff and family, had to wear a full-length yellow paper step-in, gloves, and a mask. Common hand sanitizer doesn't kill *C. diff*, so everyone had to scrub with soap and water. A janitor bleached my hospital room toilet every hour, and I was embarrassed every time. (Hospital cleaning staff put themselves at risk every day as they deal with bodily fluids and waste that carry all kinds of dangerous pathogens. Thank them. Be kind to them. Pay them more.)

Still, I wasn't worried. The doctors told me that *C. diff* usually goes away with a round of antibiotics and, not knowing any better, I believed them. On Christmas Eve in 2012, I was discharged to my parents' house, where I spent the following days taking vancomycin and obsessively bleaching the upstairs toilet

---

7. Pradeep Kumar Mada and Mohammed U. Alam, "Clostridium Difficile," in *StatPearls* (Treasure Island, Fla.: StatPearls Publishing, 2020), via National Center for Biotechnology Information, updated June 2020.

designated mine; my biggest fear was that I'd get my family sick. I was afraid to touch or hug anyone. I showered until the water scalded my skin and washed my clothing as hot as the machine would go.

Though I appreciated Mom's commitment to helping me get better, it was painful to stay in her home. Six years earlier, my stepdad's son had sexually assaulted me when I was seventeen and he was thirty-four. The night it happened, we'd gathered for a "family" dinner—me, Kaetlyn, her boyfriend at the time, Mom, my soon-to-be stepdad, and my soon-to-be stepbrother, Aaron. It was the second time I'd interacted with him so I didn't know him at all, but the dinner table mood was jovial and everyone seemed excited to get to know each other.

Mom and Dad's marriage—a cold and eventually violent relationship—had ended in 2001. Dad then sank further into the alcoholism that killed him when I was twenty years old, and Mom became increasingly devoted to Christianity. She didn't date after the divorce, but when she reconnected with my stepdad, a former flame, at a high school reunion, things got serious fast. His wife had recently died after a long illness. The need for companionship was coupled with the wistfulness of rekindling a youthful romance cut short when he left for the air force. Marriage was decided upon right away. My stepdad—a kind, simple man with a mind for machines and a heart for caretaking—was the opposite of Dad. He had a good job and a cute little home, so I could see why Mom felt safe with him.

At dinner, we soon-to-be siblings bonded over shared musical tastes and cracked a lot of jokes. After dinner, we went our separate ways: me to a high school party and the older siblings to a bar. Before they married, my parents split their time between my stepdad's house and Mom's house, where I lived then with

Kaetlyn and my niece, Zoe. I can't remember which house they went to that evening.

When I needed a ride after the party to Kaetlyn's boyfriend's apartment, where we'd planned to stay the night, Aaron said he was happy to pick me up. I could tell he'd been drinking when I got in the car, but I didn't say anything. Teenage girls often try to be agreeable, even in dangerous situations—a protective mechanism many of us carry into womanhood. And besides, I was used to riding in cars with drunken men like Dad. We got to the apartment, ate pizza, and went to bed: Kaetlyn and her boyfriend in the bedroom, me on one sofa, Aaron on another sofa across the room. I tucked my flip phone under my pillow, as I always did, and fell asleep.

Disoriented, I felt someone's sticky breath on my neck. Then a hand was up my shirt and under my bra. In my brain, I was trying to wake up, trying to call out, trying to reach for the phone under my pillow. Instead, I froze. Aaron's weight was on top of me. His hands were on my breasts. He was kissing and licking my neck. He reached for the zipper of my jeans but fumbled and gave up. I was silent. I closed my eyes tight and tried to keep my body stiff and cold like a statue. And then, he passed out with his full weight on top of me. I tried not to move too much—I didn't want him to wake up—but I struggled to find my cell phone. *Where the hell was it?* I needed to call Kaetlyn for help. I needed to call 911. But the phone wasn't there. (Later, I learned that Kaetlyn had come out for a glass of water and set it on the counter while I was asleep, thinking I'd be more comfortable without it under my head.) Aaron, still fully passed out, slumped off of me and onto the floor. I wanted to scream or run or find a heavy object to bash his head with. But I was frozen. I stayed awake the rest of the night—eight torturous hours—watching every movement, every breath coming from the body on the floor below me.

When Kaetlyn came out of the bedroom that morning to make us breakfast, she commented that it was odd Aaron was on the floor and not the couch. He laughed it off. I said nothing. When she drove me home, I still said nothing. But when I got in the shower, I fell to my knees and started sobbing.

"What's going on? What happened?" Kaetlyn asked, peeking through the curtain.

"I . . . I . . . I don't know (*sob*)! Aaron . . . he . . . he tried to . . . to get on me (*sob*)!" I didn't have the language to explain that I'd been sexually assaulted.

Kaetlyn wrapped me up in a towel and told me it was going to be okay, that I was safe, that I never had to see him again, that she was going to fucking murder him. I listened from the bathroom as she called Mom, screaming so hard her voice cracked. Mom said it must be a misunderstanding or that Aaron was drunk and didn't know what he was doing. Years after, around the time I moved to New York, she wrote me a letter arguing that I needed to take responsibility for "the incident" because I'd been drinking, too (one cup of keg beer at the party). Mom is a lovable person—friendly and silly, a good storyteller, the best caretaker when you're sick. Growing up, Kaetlyn's and my friends adored her. But when it came to protecting her daughters, she just . . . failed, maybe because her own trauma got in the way or maybe out of self-preservation. Either way, a few months after the assault, Mom married my stepdad with none of their children present.

To this day, my parents maintain a relationship with Aaron. Mom calls him "son." It will never stop being painful. It will never stop being hard to love my parents—it's a choice I must actively make. And that means that relying on them during health crises is all the more complicated. Long-term illness doesn't fix families. If anything, chronic illness makes the knotty webs that families weave even trickier to untangle. Mom loves me *and* she's hurt me. I want independence *and* I need my parents. As the round of antibiotics came to an end, I decided to travel back to New York again. The infection was almost gone, I thought, and I needed to get back to my work, my apartment, my life.

When I got back to New York in early January 2013, four days passed before I was in a Brooklyn emergency room with a recurrent *C. diff* infection. I started another course of vancomycin— "Sometimes it takes two rounds," the ER doctor assured me. Two weeks and another hospital stay later: another positive test. See, *C. diff* thrives in already-compromised guts, and mine was full of inflammation and ulceration from IBD—perfect nooks and crannies for bacteria to multiply. An infection that's difficult to treat even in a healthy gut became nightmarish in mine, and folks with underlying illnesses like IBD face a higher risk of death due to *C. diff*.

Thankfully, I was referred by a college acquaintance to a bright, capable gastroenterologist at Weill Cornell on the Upper East Side of Manhattan. She was the first to affirm the interrelation of my symptoms and talk to me about the mountainous mental challenges I faced with IBD and *C. diff*. She was up-to-date on new research and treatment options and suggested a fecal transplant, which she could coordinate should antibiotics fail. In reviewing my records, she wasn't convinced that I had ulcerative colitis, so she changed my diagnosis to "indeterminate

IBD." (It would be another two years before my Crohn's diagnosis.) She was the first doctor who made me feel safe, heard, and understood. Convinced that vancomycin was not going to rid me of the infection, she switched me to a stronger and even pricier antibiotic called Dificid ($3,500 for twenty pills without insurance).

From January to March 2013, I hung on through what I now think of as "the Lost Winter." I spent most of my days in close proximity to a toilet. I was afraid of passing the infection on to anyone, so I isolated as much as possible. I did little else but sleep, take Dificid, work from home, and taxi to and from doctor's appointments. Even a cab ride to the doctor's office meant taking large doses of antidiarrheal medicine to prevent accidents, but antidiarrheal medication is risky for people with *C. diff* because it traps the bacteria's toxins in the colon longer—it's actually better to pass it than to hold it. I sometimes went weeks without going outside, and as winter turned into spring, I grew increasingly unsure whether my life would ever become more than days and nights in a bathroom or bound to my bed. Mentally, I was unraveling.

CHAPTER 2

Doctors

Doctors become immediate and central characters in any chronically ill person's story. I always say that for every ten bad doctors in the United States there's one good one, and for patients I've spoken to in rural areas, this *very nonscientific* statistic becomes even more dismal. Away from urban areas, fewer practitioners exist, so there's little to no ability to switch doctors or to get a second opinion without extensive travel. Americans who live outside big cities remain stuck with whoever is geographically convenient. Telemedicine is helping this some,[1] but a large rural chunk of this country still lacks effective high-speed internet access.[2]

I live in New York City, where there's no shortage of doctors.

1. Patti Neighmond, "With Rural Health Care Stretched Thin, More Patients Turn to Telehealth," NPR, last updated July 7, 2019; accessed February 4, 2020, https://www.npr.org/sections/health-shots/2019/07/07/737618560/with-rural-health-care-stretched-thin-more-patients-turn-to-telehealth.

2. Monica Anderson, "About a Quarter of Rural Americans Say Access to High-Speed Internet Is a Major Problem," Pew Research Center, last updated September 10, 2018; accessed February 2, 2020, https://www.pewresearch.org/fact-tank/2018/09/10/about-a-quarter-of-rural-americans-say-access-to-high-speed-internet-is-a-major-problem/.

(Fun fact: Crohn's disease was discovered at New York's own Mount Sinai Hospital in 1932.) Research at the highest level takes place here, and some of the best hospitals in the world are no farther away than a cab ride. If I don't like a physician, it's simple enough for me to find a different one who accepts my insurance, for which I can afford to pay $700/month. My state's health insurance marketplace is abundant compared to most, and I can't be kicked off my plan for a preexisting condition or because my health needs are too expensive (thanks, Obama). I don't regularly use mobility aids like a walker or a wheelchair and when I'm feeling well enough, I don't have trouble getting around spaces designed for able bodies (which is almost all spaces). I'm white, so I don't deal with the dangerous racism that's prevalent in health care and that leads to worse outcomes—including death—for people, especially women, of color. *Especially* Black women. I'm thin, so I don't receive the brunt of fatphobia or have my symptoms dismissed with a wave of a hand and "you just need to lose weight." And I'm cis, so I don't avoid seeking medical care out of fear of transphobia or being misgendered. I have the privilege—more than privilege, really; I have power—in the ways I'm able to navigate the health-care system.

Moreover, IBD is considered a "first world disease." White people and people of Ashkenazic Jewish descent have a higher-than-average risk of getting IBD, and even though IBD is increasing among the Black population in the United States and the United Kingdom,[3] the public image of IBD remains white. This, unfortunately, matters when it comes to fundraising and

---

3. "African-Americans and IBD," Johns Hopkins Medicine, last modified March 3, 2016; accessed February 2, 2020, https://www.hopkinsmedicine.org/news/articles /african-americans-and-ibd.

paying for research. I will never be the most oppressed person in any room when it comes to being sick. If I had to deal with just one negative bias—leave alone overlapping geographic, racial, gender, or weight prejudices—my health outcomes would surely be worse.

This book isn't about the American health-care system and it's *entirely* about the American health-care system, because chronically ill bodies are at its mercy. Good health care allows me and people like me to live more independent, sustained lives—and in my country, in my lifetime at least, insurance has been required to access that care. Sometimes I fantasize about what it would be like to be free of the fear of losing my health insurance; how much of my brain space—of this country's collective thinking power—would be uninhibited to focus on other things? We've been fooled into thinking that basic human needs, like access to health care, are indulgences reserved for those who "worked hard enough." I know that health care is a human right and that gets me called *libtard* and *snowflake* and worse. But there's nothing radical about *not* wanting to die for lack of health insurance. What's so radical about wanting to live?

This is the part of the book where I can imagine the Amazon reviews: "Gee, I was with her until she got all *political*." This book is about my body, and I don't live in an apolitical one. Chronic illness is a justice issue. Health justice—the work I do through writing and advocacy—means not only free and accessible health care for all, but secure homes and public spaces, clean water, freedom from police violence (disabled people make up half of cop shooting victims), preventive care, environmental health, gender affirmation and care, and sexual and reproductive autonomy. As the COVID-19 pandemic and protests against police violence overlapped during the spring and summer of

2020, I saw them not as two separate issues but as two branches of the same root. Racism is a public health emergency. Health justice *is* racial justice.

Here's what it's like in the United States: First, let's remember that nearly thirty million Americans don't have health insurance at all,[4] a number that's risen for the first time in a decade thanks to cuts in public health programs like Medicaid and the Children's Health Insurance Program (CHIP). Women and children report the highest uninsured rates, and an estimated 45 percent of Americans ages nineteen to sixty-four are inadequately insured or underinsured.[5] And even for people *with* insurance, deductibles and out-of-pocket expenses often keep them from seeking care; plus, a lot of plans don't cover dental or vision because teeth and eyes in need of care and correction are, for whatever reason, considered separate from the rest of the body. And though mental health care has improved somewhat under the Affordable Care Act (ACA), one in five people with a mental health condition still aren't getting professional care.[6] Less than 50 percent of American adults with clinical depression receive treatment—this could be for a variety of factors including lack of insurance

---

4. Stephanie Armour, "Number of Uninsured Americans Rises for First Time in a Decade," *Wall Street Journal*, last modified September 10, 2019; accessed February 2, 2020, https://www.wsj.com/articles/number-of-americans-without-insurance-shows-first-increase-since2008-11568128381.

5. Sara R. Collins, Herman K. Bhupal, and Michelle M. Doty, "Health Insurance Coverage Eight Years After the ACA," Commonwealth Fund, last updated February 7, 2019; accessed February 2, 2020, https://www.commonwealthfund.org/publications/issue-briefs/2019/feb/health-insurance-coverage-eight-years-after-aca.

6. Jeanne Lee, "How to Learn if Your Insurance Covers Mental Health Treatment." Policygenius, last updated May 21, 2019; accessed February 24, 2020, https://www.policygenius.com/blog/how-to-learn-if-your-insurance-covers-mental-health-treatment/.

coverage, lack of access to mental health care, the stigma surrounding therapy and medication, or a decreased motivation to seek help.[7] And at-home health care for the chronically ill and the elderly is hard to qualify for and even harder to get insurance to cover; caregiving usually falls to the family, whether they're prepared to take it on or not.

A 2019 *American Journal of Medicine* study[8] of 9.5 million newly diagnosed cancer patients found that nearly half lose their entire life savings within two years due to out-of-pocket treatment costs, and 62 percent of cancer patients are in debt because treatment—even with insurance—is so expensive (on top of this, cancer treatment is so invasive that it requires many to stop working). A 2010 *JAMA* study of 3,721 acute myocardial infarction patients found that many delayed seeking care because of financial concerns.[9] That's right: People *in the midst of a heart attack* didn't go to the ER because they were afraid it would cost too much even with insurance. They aren't the only ones: According to a 2019 Kaiser Family Foundation poll, half of American adults said they skipped necessary health care in the last year due to cost, and one in eight said their health condition got worse as a result of missing or delaying an appointment.[10]

7. Ibid.

8. Adrienne Gilligan et al., "Death or Debt? National Estimates of Financial Toxicity in Persons with Newly-Diagnosed Cancer," *American Journal of Medicine* 131, no. 10 (2018): P1187–99.E5.

9. Kim G. Smolderen et al., "Health Care Insurance, Financial Concerns in Accessing Care, and Delays to Hospital Presentation in Acute Myocardial Infarction," *Journal of the American Medical Association* 303, no. 14 (2010): 1392–1400.

10. Ashley Kirzinger et al., "Data Note: Americans' Challenges with Health Care Costs," Kaiser Family Foundation, last updated June 11, 2019; accessed February 26, 2020, https://www.kff.org/health-costs/issue-brief/data-note-americans-challenges-health-care-costs/.

What's clear is that the private health insurance system is failing. The few people it's working for are those who profit from its lucrative costs and those who can wield it for exploitation—an insurance holder in an abusive marriage or the bad boss who leverages it against employees. A January 2020 Harvard study looking at government data between 1998 and 2017 reported that even under the ACA, "most measures of unmet need for physician services have shown no improvement, and financial access to physician services has decreased . . . [due to] narrow networks, high-deductible plans, and higher co-pays."[11] Further, the study found that the number of adults with health insurance who were unable to see a doctor rose over twenty years from 7 to 12 percent. That's a *60 percent* increase in people aged eighteen to sixty-four who can't afford to see a doctor even though they have insurance. The study's authors went on to write: "In Canada, only 1 percent of adults 45 years old or older with a chronic disease reported a cost-related unmet health need, compared to 18.7 percent in our U.S. sample." Even twenty years before the catastrophe of the COVID-19 pandemic, the United States had the most expensive health-care system in the world yet came in 72nd out of the World Health Organization's 191 member nations for the level of health that system achieved for its population.[12] Annually, forty-five thousand American deaths were associated with a lack of health insurance; that meant working-age people without insurance were at a 40 percent higher risk

11. Laura Hawks et al., "Trends in Unmet Need for Physician and Preventive Care Services in the United States, 1998–2017," *JAMA Internal Medicine* 180, no. 3 (2020): 439–48; published online January 27, 2020, https://jamanetwork.com/journals/jamainternalmedicine/article-abstract/2759743.

12. Ajay Tandon et al., "Measuring Overall Health System Performance for 191 Countries," World Health Organization, published 2000.

of death—even when taking into consideration socioeconomic factors—than the same age group with insurance.[13] And, again, even then, the life expectancy gap between rich and poor Americans was the highest it had ever been: 20 years.[14] That's right: Wealthy folks have been getting *twenty extra years* of life in large part because they can afford and access health care.

Prescription drug pricing offers an especially evil aspect to this baffling, arbitrary health-care system, making necessary drugs like insulin so expensive that patients ration, go without entirely, or rely on "black market" insulin exchanges that flourish on the internet. Five years ago, the every-six-weeks drug infusions I take to manage IBD were billed to my insurance at $15,000—now they're billed anywhere between $70,000 and $90,000 and then my infusion center and my insurance provider do some sort of backdoor negotiating over the price insurance will actually pay (all the while making me, the consumer, believe I'm costing the insurance company a whole heck of a lot more than I am). Ninety thousand dollars. *For the same medication.* I hear similar stories every day in my support groups from people who'd be nonfunctioning or dead without access to our doctors and medications. Remdesivir, an antiviral drug used in the treatment of COVID-19 patients, costs privately insured patients $3,120 for a five-day course via the drugmaker Gilead; it takes roughly $10 in raw materials to make the drug.[15]

---

13. David Cecere, "New Study Finds 45,000 Deaths Annually Linked to Lack of Health Coverage," *Harvard Gazette*, last updated September 17, 2009; accessed February 8, 2020, https://news.harvard.edu/gazette/story/2009/09/new -study-finds-45000-deaths-annually-linked-to-lack-of-health-coverage/.

14. Richard Luscombe, "Life Expectancy Gap Between Rich and Poor US Regions Is More Than 20 Years," *Guardian*, last updated May 8, 2017; accessed February 6, 2020.

15. Sydney Lupkin, "Remdesivir Priced at More Than $3,100 for a Course of Treatment," NPR Shots, published June 29, 2020; accessed July 5, 2020, https://www

It's no wonder, then, that thirty-four million people in the United States say they've lost a friend or family member due to inability to afford medical care.[16] It's a particularly American cruelty to make sick people beg for financial help via Go Fund Me while insurance CEOs rake in tens of millions of dollars every year. What filmmaker Ava DuVernay said about the criminal justice system is true for the health-care system, too: "It isn't broken. It was built this way." (If you'd like to read more about the baffling ways our health-care system functions—as it was designed to under capitalism—I recommend *An American Sickness* by Elisabeth Rosenthal.)

Some groups of people are more at risk than others. Fifty-nine percent of Health Professional Shortage Areas (HPSAs) are located in rural America.[17] These health-care-provider shortages lead to lower rates of preventive screenings, which means illnesses are caught later and become harder to treat. Less than half of all rural counties have access to obstetric services, and less than half of pregnant people in rural areas live within a thirty-minute drive from perinatal services.[18] Rural communities also report slightly higher uninsured rates than urban communities,[19] which further reduces access to care. (Not surprisingly,

---

.npr.org/sections/health-shots/2020/06/29/884648842/remdesivir-priced-at-more-than-3-100-for-a-course-of-treatment.

16. Dan Witters, "Millions in U.S. Lost Someone Who Couldn't Afford Treatment," Gallup, last updated November 12, 2019; accessed June 15, 2020, https://news.gallup.com/poll/268094/millions-lost-someone-couldnt-afford-treatment.aspx.

17. "Health Professional Shortage Area, 2017 postcard," National Conference of State Legislatures, updated June 30, 2017.

18. Peiyin Hung et al., "Access to Obstetric Services in Rural Counties Still Declining, with 9 Percent Losing Services, 2004–14," *Health Affairs* 36, no. 9 (2017).

19. Jennifer Cheeseman Day, "Rates of Uninsured Fall in Rural Counties, Remain Higher Than Urban Counties," United States Census Bureau, last updated April 9,

states that expanded Medicaid report better insured rates in their rural communities than nonexpansion states.)

Black mothers are four times more likely to die in childbirth than white mothers,[20] and this doesn't improve as income or education increases. High-profile stories in recent years highlighted these risks: Serena Williams, the most accomplished athlete of our lifetime, came close to dying after giving birth to her daughter because caretakers ignored her symptoms (and her own self-advocacy!) of a pulmonary embolism, a blood clot condition she had a history of. Beyoncé, one of the wealthiest and most famous musical artists ever, suffered from preeclampsia, a sudden, threatening rise in blood pressure that can result in seizures, and ended up having an emergency C-section. Her twins spent weeks in the NICU. The preeclampsia rate for Black women is 60 percent higher than for white women,[21] and after birth, Black infants are 2.5 times more likely to die in the first year of life than white infants.[22] An August 2020 study from George Mason University that analyzed data from 1992 through 2015 found that Black newborns were three times more likely to die in the hospital when cared for by white physicians. (That mortality rate shrank up to 58 percent when Black doctors were in

2019; accessed February 2, 2020, https://www.census.gov/library/stories/2019/04/health-insurance-rural-america.html.

20. Amy Roeder, "America Is Failing Its Black Mothers," *Harvard Public Health: Magazine of the Harvard T. H. Chan School of Public Health*, Winter 2019; accessed February 2, 2020, https://www.hsph.harvard.edu/magazine/magazine_article/america-is-failing-its-black-mothers/.

21. Kathryn Fingar et al., "Delivery Hospitalizations Involving Preeclampsia and Eclampsia, 2005–2014," Healthcare Cost and Utilization Project, Statistical Brief #222, April 2017.

22. Rogelio Saenz, "The Growing Color Divide in U.S. Infant Mortality," Population Reference Bureau, last updated October 12, 2017; accessed February 2, 2020, https://www.prb.org/colordivideininfantmortality/.

charge.) Beyond pregnancy, Black women get breast cancer at lesser rates than white women but die much more often from it.[23] Similar statistics exist for colorectal cancer, pancreatic cancer, and stomach cancer. They're also twice as likely to have a stroke versus white women, at younger ages, and with more severe aftereffects.[24] Black people in the United States are twice as likely to live without safe drinking water and three times more likely to die from air pollution–related illness.[25] Black communities suffered more than white ones from COVID-19, and even before quantities of data came in, we knew that Black patients were dying at a much higher rate than white patients. Seventy percent of people killed by COVID-19 in Chicago were Black, though the Black population makes up 29 percent of the city;[26] in Milwaukee, those statistics were 81 percent and 38 percent.[27] (If you want to learn more about the impact of socioeconomic factors on Black health, I recommend reading the

23. "Breast Cancer Rates Among Black Women and White Women," Centers for Disease Control and Prevention, last updated September 13, 2018; accessed February 2, 2020, https://www.cdc.gov/cancer/dcpc/research/articles/breast_cancer _rates_women.htm.

24. "African-American Women and Stroke," Centers for Disease Control and Prevention; accessed February 2, 2020, https://www.cdc.gov/stroke/women.htm.

25. Brentin Mock, "If You Want Clean Water, Don't Be Black in America," Bloomberg CityLab, last updated January 26, 2016; accessed February 2, 2020, https://www.citylab.com/equity/2016/01/if-you-want-clean-water-dont-be-black -in-america/426927/.

26. Elliott Ramos and María Inés Zamudio, "In Chicago, 70% of COVID-19 Deaths Are Black," WBEZ, last updated April 5, 2020; accessed April 10, 2020, https://www.wbez.org/stories/in-chicago-70-of-covid-19-deaths-are-black /dd3f295f-445e-4e38-b37f-a1503782b507.

27. Zak Cheney-Rice, "COVID-19's Racial Death Gap Was Predictable," *New York Intelligencer*, last updated April 8, 2020; accessed April 10, 2020, https:// nymag.com/intelligencer/2020/04/covid-19-hits-black-milwaukee-and-other -communities-hard.html.

racial weathering hypothesis and subsequent research.) Lupus, an autoimmune disease that attacks the body's healthy tissue, is two to three times more common among women of color and kills Black people at a three-times-higher rate than white people. And because of the COVID-related run on hydroxychloroquine, a medication used to treat lupus, patients had a harder time accessing necessary treatment.

Communities of color, particularly Black communities, suffer higher rates of and worse outcomes from asthma, which costs $80 billion a year in doctor visits, prescriptions, and missed work;[28] meanwhile, white people disproportionately create air pollution. Redlining—the economic policy that excludes Black neighborhoods from financial services, like mortgages—has been illegal on paper since the 1970s but is still associated with higher ER visits for asthma.[29] (And redlining still very much exists across sectors including health care; for example, insurance companies can participate in the ACA exchange in select areas that they've deemed "desirable."[30]) In short, Black people receive inferior health care and suffer from worse health-care outcomes than white patients, whether the illnesses are acute or chronic.

As for obese patient outcomes, obese women are less likely to seek screening for gynecological cancers for fear that doctors will

---

28. Tursynbek Nurmagambetov, Robin Kuwahara, and Paul Garbe, "The Economic Burden of Asthma in the United States, 2008–2013," *Annals of the American Thoracic Society* 15, no. 3 (2018): 348–56.

29. Kaelyn Forde, "'Redlining' Linked to Increased Asthma ER Visits: Study," *Al Jazeera News*, last updated January 29, 2020; accessed April 8, 2020, https://www.aljazeera.com/ajimpact/linked-increased-asthma-er-visits-study-200128220402878.html.

30. Phil Mattera, "Healthcare Redlining," *Facing South: The Online Magazine for the Institute for Southern Studies*, last updated February 14, 2014; accessed April 10, 2020, https://www.facingsouth.org/2014/02/healthcare-redlining.html.

discriminate against them due to their weight.[31] This often leads to later diagnoses and more-difficult-to-treat, progressive cancers; obese people suffer worse outcomes and higher rates of death across all cancers. (A note on the language here: There's movement away from using "obese" as the medical term, as it's based on the flawed body mass index, which suggests that all "obese" people are unhealthy by default. "Fat" is preferred in most body positive, body acceptance, and body neutrality circles. After all, "fat" is just a descriptor—the stigma that comes with the word has been created and reinforced by the people and corporations who profit off weight loss and fat shame. There's no more value in "thin" than "fat" when you remove what we've made of those words.) Primary care providers (PCPs) report spending less time—*28 percent less*, according to one study—with obese patients.[32] PCPs in that study also reported viewing obese patients as "more annoying" and said they felt less patience when dealing with heavier patients. A 2016 survey found that 90 percent of emergency departments lacked imaging equipment suitable for heavier patients,[33] meaning diagnostic tests aren't available for those patients suffering from strokes, blood clots, abdominal pain, and bodily trauma. Heavy patients deal with a difficult conundrum: Doctors often assume a higher weight to automatically mean "unhealthy," but at the same time, doctors overlook these patients' true health problems when neglecting to properly screen them due to weight.

---

31. S. M. Phelan et al., "Impact of Weight Bias and Stigma on Quality of Care and Outcomes for Patients with Obesity," *Obesity Reviews* 16, no. 4 (2015): 319–26.

32. Ibid.

33. Gina Kolata, "Why Do Obese Patients Get Worse Care? Many Doctors Don't See Past the Fat," *New York Times*, last updated September 25, 2016; accessed February 2, 2020, https://www.nytimes.com/2016/09/26/health/obese -patients-health-care.html.

Our health-care system is exceptionally unkind when it comes to the trans community. According to a 2015 survey of 27,715 transgender adults in the United States,[34] 23 percent reported avoiding medical care out of fear of discrimination. Thirty-three percent reported a negative experience in a medical setting, including being harassed or outright denied care. Nearly half of trans people report struggling with depression and a third report anxiety. They use drugs and alcohol at higher rates than their cis counterparts, with many reporting substance use as self-medication. Forty percent of trans people report having attempted suicide (*36 percent higher* than the rest of the population). Trans women—especially trans women of color—are disproportionately incarcerated,[35] and 1 in 4 report being denied health-care services while in jail or prison.[36] In mid-June 2020, the Trump administration rolled back health-care protections for trans people under Section 1557 of the ACA, which means providers can deny not only gender-affirming care but *all* care. An already vulnerable population will undoubtedly be hurt further should this rollback be allowed to stand. (As Adam Serwer wrote so poignantly in the *Atlantic*: For this administration, the cruelty is the point.)

All these statistics don't just materialize out of thin air. They happen because health-care teachers, texts (a 2017 report on

34. "2015 U.S. Transgender Survey," National Center for Transgender Equality, published December 2016.

35. "LGBTQ People Behind Bars: A Guide to Understanding the Issues Facing Transgender Prisoners and Their Legal Rights," National Center for Transgender Equality, published October 2018.

36. Sandy E. James et al., *The Report of the 2015 U.S. Transgender Survey* (Washington, D.C.: National Center for Transgender Equality, December 2016); accessed July 5, 2020, https://www.transequality.org/sites/default/files/docs/USTS-Full-Report-FINAL.PDF.

nursing school textbooks found Black patients listed as more likely to "report higher pain intensity than other cultures" and Jewish patients as "vocal and demanding," for example[37]), and providers can be racist, homophobic, transphobic, xenophobic, fatphobic, and misogynistic, and those prejudices result in poorer health and even death for patients. This is a systemic problem that hurts entire communities—communities that already have a difficult and painful history when it comes to health care. (See: "Tuskegee Study of Untreated Syphilis in the Negro Male," Henrietta Lacks, J. Marion Sims, forced sterilization, "Mississippi appendectomy," wet nursing, "husband stitch," diabetic amputations, homosexuality as mental illness, disparities in schizophrenia diagnoses, beliefs about Black pain tolerance, "gender identity disorder," gay blood ban, Dr. A. C. Jackson, institutionalization for physical and mental disabilities.) Sometimes this widespread abuse is less overtly violent but just as damaging. As writer Jeneen Interlandi highlighted in a piece for the Pulitzer Prize–winning "1619 Project," Black Americans were purposely excluded from the New Deal, the Social Security and Wagner Acts of 1935, the Fair Labor Standards Act of 1938, Aid to Families with Dependent Children, and the GI Bill.[38] Health insurance was harder for Black people to obtain, and when they did have health insurance, hospitals were often segregated or white-only. These exclusions negatively impacted, and continue to impact, the health of

37. Rozina Sini, "Publisher Apologizes for 'Racist' Text in Medical Book," BBC News, last updated October 20, 2017; accessed February 2, 2020, https://www.bbc.com/news/blogs-trending-41692593.

38. Jeneen Interlandi, "Why Doesn't the United States Have Universal Health Care? The Answer Has Everything to Do with Race," *New York Times Magazine*, last updated August 14, 2019; accessed February 2, 2020, https://www.nytimes.com/interactive/2019/08/14/magazine/universal-health-care-racism.html.

generations of Black families. (If you want to read more about how modern American medicine was built on the exploitation of Black people, I recommend *Medical Apartheid: The Dark History of Medical Experimentation on Black Americans from Colonial Times to the Present* by Harriet A. Washington and *Killing the Black Body: Race, Reproduction, and the Meaning of Liberty* by Dorothy Roberts.)

The health-care system, even when it functions well, is far from perfect. We're taught to trust doctors with our bodies, and sometimes abusive practitioners take advantage of that trust in the vilest ways. Doctors have publicly come under fire for rampant sexual abuse (Larry Nassar and USA Gymnastics), fertility fraud (doctors in the United States and the Netherlands used their own sperm to inseminate dozens of patients instead of chosen donor samples), and sexual assault (too many examples to list here). Once, when I was hospitalized, a [male] resident doctor came on to me so overtly during an abdominal exam, while my hospital gown was pulled up just below my breasts and my underwear rolled down to just above my pubic bone, that I cried. Another time, a nurse asked if she could pass my phone number along to her son. During my longest hospitalization in 2015, a [male] doctor called me "hysterical" for crying and sent a [male] priest to counsel me in my hospital bed. More times than I can count, physicians did not ask for consent before touching me.

I'm not arguing that all physicians are bad or have ill intentions. Lots of great doctors exist, and I still believe that most of them sincerely want to help people above all else. The American health-care system requires that providers work long hours in stressful conditions, churning through as many patients as they can like an assembly line. Patients can be demanding, unpredictable, and downright mean. Still, the burden of professionalism and gaining of trust should remain on the health-care provider—not the patient, who, in good faith, just wants to feel better.

I've been to more doctors in the last ten years than in the rest of my life combined. I've seen gastroenterologists, endocrinologists, internists, emergency physicians, pain medicine specialists, infectious disease doctors, immunologists, and gynecologists, among others. When I was initially diagnosed in 2012 with UC, the central Illinois–based gastroenterologist acted like the diagnosis was no big deal and didn't explain much about it— just that it was chronic (a word I didn't fully understand), that I needed to take four large maroon pills every day, and that I should follow up with his office. When I had the follow-up appointment, the doctor again told me the disease wouldn't affect my life. I could eat whatever I wanted (wrong), I'd be okay as long as I kept up with the medication he prescribed (wrong), and I wouldn't have to change my lifestyle (wrong). I left that appointment thoroughly confused, as all the books and online forums I'd read made IBD seem life-altering (right).

Several weeks following that appointment, when I flew to New York, only to return to Illinois soon after with Mom, a positive *C. diff* test and another hospitalization under my belt, I was back at the diagnosing GI's office to figure out what was happening. I knew I had UC and I knew I had *C. diff* because the doctors told me so, but I didn't understand. What had caused it? Why was this happening to me? How could I get better? Why was I in so much pain all the time? Kaetlyn went with me to the appointment because she could see I was fragile and needed someone else to ask the questions and take notes. She felt

I wasn't getting proper answers from the doctors I'd seen, so she stepped in to serve as my advocate.

The GI who diagnosed me wasn't in, so we saw his practice partner instead. I could tell right away that he didn't take Kaetlyn and me, then twenty-nine and twenty-four, seriously. He made a bad joke about the blessing of my disease being that I could eat Big Macs and not gain any weight ('cause I'd shit them right out, get it?). He delivered the joke as though my disease was lucky: *Don't you know women value being thin above all else?* I asked about my new symptoms: joint pain, swollen abdomen, stomach cramps so intense they left me unable to breathe. He said none of those things were connected to IBD or *C. diff.* When I began to cry uncontrollably, he blinked at me like a fish peering out of its tank. I left that appointment wondering if life with my diagnosis was worth living. It wasn't until I saw the kind, capable GI at Weill Cornell in New York that I began to make some sense of my illness. (My insurance changed and I wasn't able to see her in-network anymore, but I still recommend her to anyone who asks me for an IBD doctor.)

I chose my current gastroenterologist, whom I call "Doc," like any good millennial: He accepted my insurance, his office was within walking distance of my apartment, he had good online reviews, and, as a bonus, he was affiliated with Methodist, my preferred hospital. I was in a moderate flare-up in 2014 that needed attention before it spiraled into something worse. Neither Doc nor I had any idea then what the next couple of years had in store—flares, impactions, recurrent *C. diff,* two more fecal transplants, *E. coli* infection, sepsis—but I'm forever thankful that proximity and a five-star Yelp page brought us together.

One thing you should know about Doc is that he's tall. Like six and a half feet tall. When we hug—because we're that friendly now—my head meets his chest. His wide shoulders take up space in a room and people pay attention when he talks. He speaks with a soft Lebanese accent that makes words—even ones like *colonoscopy* and *inflammation*—sound melodic. Doc does not give or take bullshit. But he's also quick to smile and laugh—sometimes when he gets to belly laughing, his eyes crinkle up and all his teeth show, so I can imagine what he looked like as a kid, taller than his friends. Doc takes calls and texts from his patients at all hours. He's always stepping out of the room to explain a test result or medication to someone. (I often wonder just how many people have his cell phone number.)

Doc poses thoughtful questions and listens intently when I answer. When it's my turn to ask, he answers thoroughly and is always saying, "Does that make sense?" to be sure I get it. He never makes me feel rushed, which I appreciate because I ask probably *too many* questions. When he needs to do exams of any kind, he tells me first what they entail from start to finish and asks for consent. When I say no to exams (and I do), he doesn't shame me—he finds another solution. We agree on treatment plans together, and I always leave our appointments with action to take, which makes me feel more in control of my illness. In our conversations over the years, I learned that Doc's wife is also a gastroenterologist and that she has UC. She had to take a year away from medical school because of her illness, and witnessing the effects of her illness made Doc become a GI instead of a surgeon. Though he can't understand what it's like to live with the disease himself, he sees how it affects the person closest to him, and that makes him more understanding and compassionate with his patients. It's personal for him.

During my long hospitalization in the spring of 2015, Doc checked on me most evenings before he went home even though the hospital was way out of his commute. He would pull up a chair next to my bed and listen while I cried. Sometimes, he would put his hand on top of mine and promise not to let anything bad happen to me. Doc met with my attending doctors and reviewed my charts and treatment plans. He gave Mom his cell phone number and told her to call or text day or night, something she took advantage of often. He consulted with other doctors and experts about my case and reported back to me about what he'd learned. Perhaps most important, when I had recurrent *C. diff* in 2015, Doc sought out Dr. G., the specialist who agreed to perform a fecal transplant when no one else would due to strict FDA regulations. Both of them fought hard for me to get the proper treatment, and it's no exaggeration that I'd be dead without the two of them.

For a while, I believed that the bad doctors I'd had were location-based: Who but the worst doctors would end up practicing in some nowhereville, anyway? It was a snobby, shortsighted opinion that I quickly learned wasn't true. Bad doctors are everywhere, even in the largest and greatest cities in the world. Though I found excellent, progressive care in New York City, I also encountered doctors who dismissed my pain, doctors who didn't listen, and doctors who flirted and acted inappropriately. I had nurses who told me my disease was caused by diet, nurses who left me without care for hours, and nurses who treated me like nothing more than an opiate seeker.

My experience as a patient, together with my years as a health journalist and the stories I've heard via support groups, helped me come up with these guidelines for what makes a good doctor (in other words, these are the things you should keep in mind as you choose a physician). When you have a chronic illness, a doctor isn't someone you see once or twice a year when you need a physical or come down with a bug. They are a central part of your life now, and they will play a major role in how well you live with your illness. You will see them often—more often than you'd care to, if we're being honest—so you need to trust and respect them. In an ideal situation, you will even *like* your doctor! But in turn, they need to meet several qualifications:

- A good doctor respects you.

To respect someone means to value their wants, needs, and rights—and though it seems like that should be common sense for any doctor, it isn't. A good physician will take time to listen to you thoroughly, without judgment, even if you're "emotional." They should ask questions that dig deeper into your health history and symptoms, filling in any gaps of information that might help them treat you. Sometimes these conversations get sensitive, and you never have to answer a question that makes you feel uncomfortable. But a good doctor should create an environment in which you know you're safe to share.

Your doctor should not make you feel stupid or behave as though they're smarter than you because you're [fill in the blank: a woman, a minority, poor, etc.]. They should always take your concerns seriously and *never* pass symptoms off as "anxiety" or "you're just stressed" without due diligence. Could it be stress or anxiety? Sure, but that's also an easy way to dismiss serious physical symptoms. And even if it is "just" stress, it's flippant to send a patient along as though that isn't also a real health concern. Along those lines, a doctor should never present weight loss as a panacea for your health concerns. And they shouldn't doubt the level of pain you're in just because you're not writhing around on the floor; chronic illness patients learn to live with a shocking amount of physical discomfort and often go about it looking natural.

Physicians should always—with *no* exceptions—honor your name and pronouns, even if they differ from what's on your identification or medical records. If you don't want to be weighed or you need to step on the scale backward to avoid seeing the reading, they should accommodate your request. If there are certain places on your body or ways that you do not want to be touched, they must comply with your needs. *Your needs come first.*

- A good doctor explains what they're going to do and why, and they ask for consent before proceeding.

One of the worst parts of chronic illness is that you feel like your body no longer belongs to you. Part of this comes from a loss of control due to the disease itself, and part of it stems from the constant poking, scanning, testing, and measuring. Chronic illness requires so many procedures, not only to get an initial diagnosis but also to monitor and manage the disease: colonoscopies, endoscopies, X-rays, CT scans, MRIs, EKGs, ultrasounds, blood tests, genetic tests, stool tests, rectal exams, pelvic exams, abdominal exams, surgeries. The list goes on and on.

These things are uncomfortable enough, but when you don't know why you're getting a certain test or exam or what's going to happen during it, it can be agonizing. A good physician explains why you need said procedure and how it will go. What parts of my body are involved and why? Will it be painful? How long will it take? Will it require any kind of anesthesia, and do I have a choice? Do I need to prep beforehand? What will the results show, and how long will it take to get them back? How will the results be delivered? Will it require follow-up testing? Does my insurance cover the cost? Are there any alternatives to this test?

When those questions have been answered, a good doctor asks if it's okay to proceed. They'll use language like: "Is it all right if I [touch here, do this exam, etc.]?"; "Can I tell you more about [this procedure, why this is important, etc.]?"; "Let me know if you feel unsure or uncomfortable"; and "Tell me at any time if you'd like to stop." You should feel comfortable saying no or asking for a few minutes to compose yourself before proceeding, knowing that your doctor will accommodate your needs. Unfortunately, there are times when you need the test or exam even when you don't want it. (Who *wants* a colonoscopy?) But a good doctor works with you to guarantee you're as comfortable as possible throughout, and that you're informed before, during, and after.

- A good doctor knows their limits.

Listen, egos exist in every profession (hello journalism, my old friend), but they're more prevalent in some than others. Medicine is one of those professions, and for good reason: These people took a shitload of tests, paid hundreds of thousands of dollars in tuition, and spent, like, fifty more years in school than the rest of us. Their jobs require a level of critical thinking and skill that many do not. Some of that ego is warranted! But it also gets in the way, and that costs the patient.

A good doctor is never too proud to ask for a second opinion or seek out an expert when a patient's care goes beyond their scope of knowledge. A good doctor knows that there's no shame in *not* knowing, and they put the needs of the patient above protecting their self-esteem. When a case gets complicated, they should be willing to collaborate with other doctors and seek out experts who know what they don't. Bottom line: A good doctor puts the patient's well-being above all else, always.

- A good doctor makes the most of their time.

Doctors work long hours, packing in as many patients as they can because that's what our health-care system demands. By some estimates, primary care physicians spend fifteen minutes or less with each patient, and research shows that this kind of time stress leads to physician burnout as well as worse patient outcomes.[39] Further research shows that on average, patients get just eleven seconds to explain their symptoms before their doctor interrupts them. Physicians are trying to make the most of their time, perhaps, but how much can they really understand about a patient in eleven seconds?[40] A short appointment might be unavoidable, but a good doctor makes the most of the time they have with their patient and maximizes the out-of-office time by ordering tests, exams, etc. If they run out of time with a patient, a good doctor will call the patient later to be sure all their questions were answered.

No matter how long or short an appointment, you should leave feeling that your questions were answered—or if they weren't, that you've been referred to a specialist who *can* answer them—and that you know what needs to happen next. You shouldn't

39. Roni Caryn Rabin, "15-Minute Visits Take a Toll on the Doctor-Patient Relationship," *Kaiser Health News*, last updated April 21, 2014; accessed February 2, 2020, https://khn.org/news/15-minute-doctor-visits/.

40. Ospina, Naykky Singh, et al., "Eliciting the Patient's Agenda," *Journal of General Internal Medicine* (2018), https://pubmed.ncbi.nlm.nih.gov/29968051/.

be more confused after a doctor's appointment than before. And you should *never* leave an appointment feeling hopeless.

- A good doctor is kind to their staff.

This is important not only for nurses, techs, and receptionists, who deserve a boss who respects them, but also for patients. Simply put, when staffers are respected, things function better: Appointments run on time, tests get ordered and completed, follow-up happens as it should, etc. Maybe this is selfish, but I want to go to a doctor's office with, for lack of a scientific term, a *good vibe*, where I can tell that morale is high and that the people who work there don't hate their jobs, where there's rapport between physician and staff, where the doctor speaks highly of the others in the office and they do the same in return. When you're a professional patient, you become a fly on the wall in hospitals and doctors' offices, and you overhear *everything*. It's easy to tell when a doctor treats their staff badly—and is that the kind of doctor you want taking care of you?

- A good doctor looks at you as a human, not an opportunity.

This should go without saying, but a good doctor sees a patient as an individual person to be treated accordingly, not as a financial opportunity. Doctors maintain relationships with the pharmaceutical industry—this is unavoidable because of the way our system functions—but it's up to a physician how closely they work with Big Pharma and how handsomely they'll profit from it. If a doctor is doling out the same medication to every patient, regardless of the specifics of their illness, you can guess that that doctor is benefiting from writing those prescriptions.

While it's illegal to receive kickbacks for writing scripts, it's not illegal for pharmaceutical companies to pay doctors as "consultants" or "speakers," and it isn't illegal for pharma reps to give gifts, trips, charitable donations, or meals to doctors and their staff as a nudge in the direction of the drug or device they represent.

Open Payments, a federal database established under the Affordable Care Act to monitor the flow of pharma industry money, found that two-thirds of Americans who'd visited a doctor in the last year saw a physician who had received money or gifts—but only 5 percent of patients were aware that their physician received those benefits. You can look up your own doctors by name at OpenPaymentsData.CMS.gov.

I've also found that every good doctor I've been to has a personal stake in the medicine they practice. This isn't a requirement when choosing a doctor, but I do think it changes the kind of care you're going to receive. Doc's wife has ulcerative colitis. The doctor who performed my first fecal transplant in 2013 lost his father to colon cancer. Dr. G., the specialist who did my second and third fecal transplants, told me he chose gastroenterology after watching different specialists during medical school: "The GIs appeared more friendly, empathetic, intuitive, and engaging." Good doctors see their loved ones in their patients; they make choices for their patients that they would make for their own family. Asking a doctor, "Why did you choose this line of medicine?" will reveal a lot about what drives them and how they view their patients.

- A good doctor communicates clearly.

Some doctors have a better bedside manner than others, a warmth and ease that make it a pleasure to speak with them.

Not all doctors maintain this ability, but that alone doesn't mean they're bad at their job. Lots of things go into communication—fluency, body language, social cues, etc.—and a doctor can still be good without having all of these perfected. It would be gross to disqualify a doctor just because they don't make impeccable eye contact, for example. What's more important is that a doctor communicates clearly, in a way that's easy for you to understand. Maybe you're a visual learner and you need your doctor to provide graphs or charts that explain your treatment. Maybe you need detailed statistical breakdowns about side effects, or you like to read double-blind studies. "Explain this to me like I'm five years old" usually works when something is going over my head. Whichever way you take in information best, that's how your doctor should communicate. And if conversations with your doctor leave you more confused than informed, it might be time to look for a new one.

- A good doctor is up-to-date on research and treatment.

It shouldn't be the patient's burden to educate their doctor. Part of a physician's job is to stay on top of research in their field, as well as new treatment options—and not just the ones peddled by drug reps. Disease research is evolving and new drugs get approved all the time; I can count a handful of treatments approved for my disease in the last decade. Individuals' chronic illnesses change over time, too—symptoms go away or new ones show up and bodies stop responding to medications that they once did. Diseases aren't treated the same way today as they were even fifteen or twenty years ago. Doctors need to know how to navigate all these changes and how to guide their patients through them.

- A good doctor acknowledges the connection between physical and mental health.

Your doctor should bring up the importance of mental health care as part of chronic illness management, and I'd be suspicious of those who don't acknowledge how depression and anxiety are connected to—I'd even argue *normal symptoms of*—chronic physical illness. A good doctor will help you navigate the mental health side of long-term illness just as they would the physical, and they should be able to refer you to a mental health professional who understands the burden of chronic illness for therapy and, if necessary, medication.

- A good doctor sides with the patient, not the insurance company.

Insurance providers don't love chronically ill people. We're expensive, we're always switching or adding new treatments, and we're hospitalized a lot. Because of this, insurance companies are always looking for ways to cut our costs through denying medications or referrals to specialists. A good doctor goes to bat for their patients and appeals the insurance company's decision if it's not in their patient's favor. Insurance companies are banking on physicians *not* appealing their decisions, so when they do, they relent more often than not. Insurance companies tell patients "no" in hopes they won't fight—but you must *always* fight. Keep pushing until you get to yes. It's cruel to make sick people plead for the care they need, but such is the American system. My three best words of advice for being chronically ill in the United States are: appeal, appeal, appeal.

Further, doctors and their staff often know about financial

assistance that insurance companies don't readily advertise. For example, I needed an expensive blood test that had to be processed by one specific lab. Insurance wasn't going to cover much of the cost, but Doc gave me a financial hardship form that reduced my out-of-pocket cost to almost nothing. Doctors' offices often have savings cards that reduce the cost of prescription drugs, sometimes down to as little as $5, even for expensive medications. It's always worth asking your doctor if they have financial assistance available.

- A good doctor is a woman.

I'm not saying this just because women are better and smarter (which *we are*). Hear me out! The research backs this up: In a twenty-year study of half a million heart attack patients, mortality rates were lower for women *and* men when the physician was a woman.[41] Women patients treated by male doctors fared the worst. Similarly, a Harvard study of 1.5 million Medicare patients found that they were less likely to die or be readmitted to the hospital when treated by a woman doctor.[42] Why? Because, according to the research, women doctors take more time to listen to their patients and they're less likely to disbelieve their patients' symptoms. I'm not saying all male doctors are lousy—my current doctors are all men and they're wonderful

---

41. Brad N. Greenwood, Seth Carnahan, and Laura Huang, "Patient–Physician Gender Concordance and Increased Mortality Among Female Heart Attack Patients," *Proceedings of the National Academy of Sciences of the United States of America* 115, no. 34 (2018): 8569–74, published August 6, 2018.

42. Yusuke Tsugawa et al., "Comparison of Hospital Mortality and Readmission Rates for Medicare Patients Treated by Male vs Female Physicians," *JAMA Internal Medicine* 177, no. 2 (2017): 206–13, published January 2017.

and I love them. The lesson here isn't to choose a doctor on gender alone but to choose a doctor who listens and takes your concerns seriously.

• Okay, so how do you find one of these good doctors?

One of the first things I tell any newly diagnosed chronically ill person to do, if they ask for my advice, is to join a support group for their specific illness. The internet makes this easier than ever for us folks who don't always feel well enough to go to an in-person meeting. Support groups are helpful for all kinds of things, one of which is asking for a doctor recommendation. Posts like this happen every day in my online IBD support group: "Can anyone recommend a gastroenterologist in the Cleveland area who takes Blue Cross/Blue Shield?" It gets dozens of responses!

The internet has also made information about doctors more available than ever. You can find out where they studied, what they specialize in, and what research they've published. As mentioned earlier, you can use Open Network to uncover how much they're benefiting from the pharmaceutical industry; you can also see if they have any serious complaints or disciplinary actions on their public record. For most physicians, you can read patient reviews that offer insight into bedside manner, communication style, and even office wait times. If you're beholden to in-network doctors, work backward: Get the list of doctors in your network, then do some internet sleuthing to decide who might be the best fit for you. It's worth calling the office to see if they offer free or low-cost consultations as well, so you can meet with—or at least speak on the phone with—potential candidates before deciding on one.

This isn't a necessity, but I also recommend finding a doctor who's affiliated with a teaching hospital. Teaching hospitals, sometimes called university hospitals, are connected to medical schools and used to train medical students and residents. Teaching hospitals focus on conducting and publishing research, are better equipped to handle rare diseases and complex cases, and cater to more diverse populations. Recent studies show that the out-of-pocket cost for patients is no higher at teaching hospitals than nonteaching hospitals. (Wait times might be longer, though.)

When you've scheduled an appointment with the doctor you've chosen, you should come prepared. Draft a list of all of your symptoms and a list of questions you want to ask the doctor, not just about your illness but about the doctor's experience and approach. It can be hard to remember things when you're not feeling well—pain takes up a lot of brainpower. If you're really sick, it can be helpful to bring a loved one along to serve as a second brain and make sure all your questions get answered. And always ask about any follow-up appointments or exams/procedures that need to be scheduled.

Here's another tip: If a health-care provider makes a choice you disagree with, ignores symptoms you bring up, or seems negligent, tell them to put it in your chart. Say you've requested more testing for abdominal pain, but the physician says it's nothing more than stress and won't proceed further. Tell them to write in your chart that they're denying further care. If there's a paper trail, it usually inspires the provider to be more diligent. This has worked time and time again in my chronic illness circles. Paper is your proof.

Now I hope this never happens, but say you experience an unprofessional or abusive doctor. What action can you take? I've outlined your options and what to expect from the process in

Appendix I, titled "Reporting a Doctor." Flip to it in the back of the book to learn more.

It is more difficult than it should be to find a good doctor under the constraints of miserly health insurance companies, but it isn't impossible. Lean on your chronically ill community for recommendations and guidance and use the good ol' internet to research. Know what qualities and qualifications to look for in a physician and understand the steps to take should a physician become unprofessional or abusive.

Searching for a doctor who suits all of your needs feels exhausting when you're managing everything else that chronic illness throws at you, but finding good care is one of the most important ways you can live well with chronic illness. In many ways, your doctor determines the quality of life you'll live with incurable/long-term illness, as they're the one guiding your treatment. You have to trust and rely on them. We have only so much control over our unpredictable, forever-sick bodies. But we do have control over who we choose to care for them.

CHAPTER 3

The Most Important Poop of Your Life

From my homebound "Lost Winter" of 2013, a February journal entry reads: *"These days are about waiting for sleep. Waking, waiting."*

Another from February: *"I remember Dad telling me about a hospital stint in the '70s when he was fighting food-borne hepatitis. According to him, the doctors predicted he'd be there for weeks. He said he meditated for three days and got to go home. Now, I have no idea if this is true or not—Dad was fond of fantasy and exaggeration. But it has me wondering: Could I harness the power of my mind to rid my body of what ails it?"*

Another: *"No one prepares you for the isolation of sickness."*

From March 9: *"I feel I've finally come undone. Unraveling like cheap thread, piling onto myself . . ."*

By March, I'd taken two more rounds of Dificid yet was still positive for *C. diff.* The bacteria destroyed my insides while the months of heavy-duty antibiotics further damaged my immune system. See, the immune cells that live in the gut make up the biggest part of the body's defense force. As Emeran Mayer, MD, wrote in *The Mind-Gut Connection*, "In other words, there are more immune cells living in the wall of your gut than circulating in our blood or residing in your bone marrow."[1] But the work of those cells is disrupted by long-term antibiotic use. While the antibiotic's goal was to get rid of the bad bacteria, it also got rid of my good bacteria—the stuff that helps fight infection and keeps the microbiome healthy.

My gastroenterologist knew I was deteriorating, and the only chance at recovery was to repopulate my colon with healthy bacteria.

I needed a fecal transplant.

The idea is simple: Poop from a healthy person is mixed with saline and transplanted via colonoscopy, endoscopy, or nasogastric tube to the gut of an unhealthy person. During and after a successful fecal transplant, the flora from the healthy stool populates the unhealthy gut with diverse bacteria, overtakes the nasty *C. diff* bacteria, and rebalances the microbiota. (A note on language: *Microbiota* are the microbes that live in the gut. One hundred trillion of them reside in the digestive tract, with the highest population in the colon. They do everything from aiding in digestion and metabolism to regulating the immune system, and they're in constant communication with the nervous system. No wonder the gut gets the nickname "the second brain." *Microbiome* is the genetic material of those microbes. The bacteria that populate the gut contain millions of genes, which, in addition to the microbes elsewhere in your body, make the genetic information we carry around 99 percent microbial![2])

---

1. Emeran Mayer, *The Mind-Gut Connection* (New York: HarperCollins, 2016), 11.

2. Michael Pollan, "Some of My Best Friends Are Germs," *New York Times Magazine*, May 15, 2013.

Fecal microbiota transplants have gotten a lot of attention in the last several years, but the "technology" is old—the first medically recorded FMT dates to the 1950s. These days, a donation is sourced from a known donor or from an anonymous stool bank like the nonprofit OpenBiome, which maintains a rigorous approval process for its donors. Under doctor supervision, freeze-dried stool capsules can be ordered online for about $2,000 before insurance.

FMT is a relatively cheap, simple, abundant, and highly effective treatment against C. diff—approximately 80 to 90 percent of C. diff patients are cured with one FMT, according to recent studies, and that cure rate goes up even further with more than one FMT.[3] Meanwhile, between 20 and 35 percent of C. diff patients fail antibiotic treatment, and 40 to 60 percent will experience a recurrent infection.[4] A study published in the New England Journal of Medicine in January 2013 found that thirteen out of sixteen people treated with fecal transplants were cured of C. diff and two of the remaining three were cured with a second transplant.[5] The results were so impressive that the researchers found it unethical to continue the control group on antibiotics, and they received transplants as well.

My gastroenterologist at Weill Cornell coordinated the FMT alongside the doctor who would perform the procedure, another

3. Lawrence J. Brandt, "Fecal Transplantation for the Treatment of Clostridium difficile Infection," Gastroenterology & Hepatology 8, no. 3 (2012): 191–94.

4. Roy J. Hopkins and Robert B. Wilson, "Treatment of Recurrent Clostridium difficile Colitis: A Narrative Review," Gastroenterology Report 6, no. 1 (2018): 21–28, published online December 18, 2017; accessed July 4, 2020, https://www .ncbi.nlm.nih.gov/pmc/articles/PMC5806400/.

5. Els van Nood et al., "Duodenal Infusion of Donor Feces for Recurrent Clostridium difficile," New England Journal of Medicine 368 (2013): 407–15, published January 31, 2013.

GI at the same hospital whose research focused on infectious disease. He'd just started doing fecal transplants then, mostly for old folks with *C. diff*; at twenty-four, I was one of the youngest patients he'd treated. (Today, he estimates that he's done at least two hundred FMTs.) He suggested I find a donor who was healthy, my same sex, close to my age, under the age of sixty-five, and antibiotic-free for at least six months. Mom had recently taken antibiotics, my stepdad was too old, Kaetlyn was pregnant with her third child (there's no ban on pregnant people donating, but it isn't recommended as pregnancy's changes on the gut flora are not well understood), and I was too embarrassed to ask anyone else. But the stakes were high, and I'd already secured a hard-to-get transplant appointment for April 2013. My niece, Zoe, a few weeks from turning nine years old then, was the only candidate. (She would also become the youngest stool donor in Weill Cornell's history.)

Kaetlyn was a twenty-one-year-old cosmetology school student when she got pregnant with Zoe. I was fifteen, a sophomore in high school. Kaetlyn interrupted my afternoon chemistry class to show me the sonogram. "It's a girl!" she yelled as she pulled me from the classroom to the hallway, where we jumped up and down, squealing and hugging. It felt like I was getting a little sister rather than a niece. When Kaetlyn gave birth in April 2004, which required Pitocin inducement and several hours of labor, I was the first family member Zoe saw, hovering wide-eyed above the warming table. We've been cosmically linked ever since. Zoe is—and always has been—curious and funny and smart and brave. As a toddler, she had all these -isms, like "wallard" for water, "pal melish" for nail polish, "strawbirdies" for strawberries, and "Danna" for grandma. We thought they were just cute little quirks until we found out she had been born with sensorineural hearing loss that required hearing aids. You would never know about her disability upon meeting her—she lip-reads so effortlessly and constantly adapts to the world around her. Sixteen years old now, Zoe is set on being a neurosurgeon and with her wild—frightening sometimes—ambition and perfect grades, I think she'll do whatever she decides to do.

My senior year of high school, Kaetlyn and Zoe moved out of our shared house—a crooked three-bedroom with a purple front door and a subprime mortgage that, with help from her siblings, Mom bought just before Zoe arrived—and settled into their own little home, a cute apartment in a complex with a walking trail, a community pool, and a duck pond. Mom began dating my stepdad and spent most nights at his house. Kaetlyn's government benefits went with her and Zoe, so the blocks of cheese and bags of cereal I relied on for many meals disappeared. Unopened bills piled up in boxes below Mom's bed, as if they would go away so long as she didn't open the envelopes. The grass grew tall and the bank took back the house. But for a moment in time, that shared house had been full of hope. We were a family there, the four of us.

When I needed the fecal transplant, Kaetlyn sat Zoe down to explain why she was the ideal choice and explained how dire the situation was. At first, Zoe refused. She cried and screamed that she wasn't going to do it. "When you're nine years old and you find out you have to poop into a bag and that poop has to go into your aunt, that's *kiiiiiind* of a weird thing," Zoe recently told me. (Now, she's also taller than I am and old enough to drive.) She laughed as she recounted the story to me at Mom's kitchen table. "I didn't realize the severity of it." Plus, everything is embarrassing when you're nine. But she soon understood that I might not recover without the transplant, and that she was the best (and only) one for the job. "I felt proud, knowing that I was doing something important for someone—someone I care about so much," Zoe said, "even if it was sort of weird."

She carried a burden heavier than any nine-year-old should: First, she'd need blood and stool tests to verify she could donate. She hollered and thrashed around so fiercely at the blood draw that nurses had to restrain her. (Kaetlyn later sent flowers and an "I'm sorry" card to the staff.) Then, she'd have to fly to New York with her mom and "Danna" and take the most important dump of her life, which would be collected, taken to the hospital, mixed with saline, and transplanted into my large intestine. She was understandably scared of the whole process, but most of all she was afraid that her poop "wouldn't save me."

Before the transplant, I had to gather supplies: colonoscopy prep to clear my bowels for the procedure; Imodium to help me hold in the transplanted stool mixture as long as possible after the procedure; and—this isn't a joke—a blender. The hospital staff asked for the sample—as fresh as possible, they requested—to be brought in a blender so they could minimize their own poop handling and cut down on the procedure's ick factor. I ordered one online after reading countless reviews for how well it handled smoothies and protein shakes. I wasn't going to risk buying a subpar blender when my life was on the line, you know? (Now that Weill Cornell uses stool from OpenBiome, there's no need for patients to find a donor or buy a blender.)

April rolled around. Zoe, Mom, and six-months-pregnant Kaetlyn, suffering from hyperemesis gravidarum—a kind of extreme morning sickness that caused her nine miserable months of nausea and vomiting—made it to New York despite one canceled and one rescheduled flight. (The first plane was struck by lightning—how's that for a bad omen?) We stayed at Weill

Cornell's "hospital hotel," an apartment-style building for patients' families, with me in one room and them in another. The rooms looked like any long-term business hotel—kitchenettes and bad watercolors—but they smelled like a hospital's telltale mix of cleaning products and decay. Zoe brought me a cobalt-blue paper crane that she'd made "for good luck"; it sits on my desk as I write this.

Kaetlyn tried to make the trip fun and less scary for Zoe by going to Times Square and the Met. She and Zoe took pictures under the New Year's Eve ball and in front of Van Gogh's *Sunflowers*. They ordered in giant plates of pasta and slices of pizza in hopes that those foods would help Zoe "go." During our conversation at Mom's kitchen table, Zoe admitted thinking, "We're in this amazing city and all I'm going to do is *poop*?" ("I would have made that child drink black coffee and smoke a cigarette if that's what it took!" Kaetlyn joked.) Meanwhile, Mom stayed close to our lodgings in case of emergency and I drank the colonoscopy prep, waiting for cramps to signal it was time to spend several hours on the toilet, until whatever I passed was clear as water. We all slept poorly that night.

The next morning, Mom called to announce that the "sample" was ready to go, and "the healthiest turd she'd ever seen." Zoe was relieved that her job was over. She and Kaetlyn stayed behind to rest while Mom, tightly clutching the blender box like a chest of precious jewels, walked a city block to the surgical center with me. I was so tired and so nervous that my legs shook, but as we continued, I got to giggling and couldn't stop.

"What if we get mugged right now," I said, "and the thief gets home to find a giant turd in a blender?"

We laughed until we cried.

Mom passed the box along to a nurse and went to the waiting

room. She flashed the ASL sign for "I love you," a gesture we'd done since my childhood. I changed into a hospital gown with familiar blue plaid and rolled to my left side on the surgical bed. As the anesthesiologist inserted the IV and told me to count backward from 10, tears rolled from the corners of my eyes. "This *has* to work," I whispered, before passing into black.

The GI spent an hour snaking the colonoscopy scope through my colon, spraying my diseased guts with the magical poop mixture. While he was in there, he took photos and biopsies that showed significant damage but not enough to warrant bowel resection or removal. Back at the "hotel," I cried—this time out of relief. My biggest fear then, besides getting someone else sick, was that my colon would be too far gone and have to be removed. I wasn't ready to live with an ostomy yet—I hadn't come to terms, after half a year of illness, with what "chronic" would mean for me, let alone the prospect of a lifetime with a waste-collecting ostomy bag. (My ostomy-related fears disappeared over time as I met dozens of IBD patients whose lives were saved by the surgery, and who credit their bags with giving them their lives back.)

The morning after the transplant, I felt physically stronger somehow, or maybe it was a renewed sense of optimism fueling the spring in my step. I was ravenously hungry for the first time in months, and Mom watched wide-eyed as I inhaled a plate of diner eggs and sausage. From December to April, food had tasted bad and had caused massive amounts of pain. I either didn't eat at all or, because I was too sick to grocery shop, ate whatever the drugstore next to my apartment offered: beef jerky, potato chips, gummy candy. It didn't need to inspire me, it just needed to provide calories to count against everything I was puking up and shitting out.

On the walk back to the hospital hotel from the diner, Mom

and I passed by Sotheby's auction house. Her face lit up as she scanned the banners advertising an open-to-the-public gem and jewelry show inside. Mom has always been a magpie with an appreciation for all things sparkly. We could never afford fine jewelry, but she loved to bead her own necklaces and find statement earrings at discount stores, dangling gold-fill florals and beaded chandeliers. Costume jewelry inherited from her mother and mother-in-law are among her most prized possessions, not because they're worth anything but because she loves the idea of an old lady (herself, someday) covered in topaz and vermeil. Inside the exhibit, Mom marveled at the giant yellow diamond solitaires and Art Deco tiaras. A Sotheby's employee saw her admiring a deep-blue sapphire cuff bracelet and took it out of the case so she could put it on. I couldn't believe that one day prior someone else's shit was being sprayed all over my insides, and today I was watching Mom giddily try on a $75,000 bracelet.

Within forty-eight hours of the procedure, I felt markedly better: My taste for food returned, my abdominal pain subsided to a dull throb, my bowel movements began to solidify (do you know the massive relief that comes from seeing a semisolid poop after months of nothing but intestinal sludge?), and my consuming fatigue started to lift. It seemed too good to be true.

You might be wondering why, given the clinical evidence that fecal transplants are the most effective treatment, they aren't the first line of defense against *C. diff* over antibiotics. The simple answer? Capitalism. Drug companies can't patent or profit from human feces, but they *can* make vancomycin and Dificid exorbitantly expensive. Even more challenging, the FDA keeps trying to regulate stool as a drug, which requires doctors to complete investigational new drug (IND) applications before they're allowed to do a transplant, delaying lifesaving treatment.

But the more complicated answer is that doctors know exactly what's in the antibiotics that treat *C. diff.* Stool, on the other hand, has countless variables: fungi, good and bad bacteria, protozoa, viruses. No two people have the same gut microbiota, and with that many unknowns comes risk. Doctors have to decide if the danger of *not* performing the transplant outweighs going through with it. For someone like me with inflammatory bowel disease, which increases the chance of *C. diff* mortality, and who'd failed round after round of antibiotics, it was worth it.

In 2019, the FDA halted an unspecified number of FMT clinical trials after one death and one invasive infection; the FDA wouldn't offer many details other than both patients were immune compromised and the stool they received was from the same donor.[6] The donor's stool contained a drug-resistant strain of *E. coli*, and whatever screening was done didn't catch that specific pathogen. Now, patients fear that the FDA will crack down on stool banks like OpenBiome, making transplant material harder to access and handing more power to for-profit drug companies. Plus, if the FDA decides not to approve the procedure—or regulates it into oblivion—insurance companies will be less willing to cover the cost, leaving more patients with an out-of-pocket burden. I was lucky enough to have excellent employer-based insurance, first at Lifehacker in 2013 and again at the *Daily Beast* in 2015, for all three of my FMTs, paying ultimately next to nothing.

It's already so difficult to access a proper transplant that some desperate patients try DIY versions. There are dozens of online forums and social media groups dedicated to guiding

6. Denise Grady, "Fecal Transplant Is Linked to a Patient's Death, the F.D.A. Warns," *New York Times*, last updated June 13, 2019; accessed February 2, 2020, https://www.nytimes.com/2019/06/13/health/fecal-transplant-fda.html.

others through the risky at-home process. There's also chatter of a potential *C. diff* vaccine in development via Pfizer,[7] but there's no telling if or when it will be on the market, or who it will be marketed to (the trial is focused on patients aged fifty and up). And of course, "microbiome therapy" start-ups have begun to pop up, seeking to profit from the exchange of human flora and gain favor with the FDA as FMT clinical trials explode for everything from depression to autism.

Fecal transplants not only work consistently but, in most cases, quickly. Though research suggests that the gut's microbiota adapts and changes for months post-FMT, symptoms can remedy within days. Through the rest of the spring and into the summer, my insides bloated, gurgled, and moved constantly. I imagined them rebuilding, like ants reconstructing a stepped-on hill. With a negative test showing the infection gone, I wondered what it would be like to live with *just* IBD. I'd contracted *C. diff* so soon after the diagnosis that I couldn't picture day-to-day life without it. My doctors warned me that *C. diff* could return in patients who've had it, especially in patients like me with underlying disease. I buried their warning somewhere deep in my brain, unable to think about going through it a second time. But two years later, *C. diff* came for me again—bringing me the closest to death I've ever been.

7. "Clostridium difficile Vaccine Efficacy Trial," Pfizer, last updated January 28, 2020; accessed March 2, 2020, https://www.pfizer.com/science/find-a-trial/nct03090191.

CHAPTER 4

Our Grief

In *The Year of Magical Thinking*, Joan Didion wrote, "Grief turns out to be a place none of us know until we reach it." Grief is different than any other feeling. Maybe it's a bunch of feelings jumbled together in a confusing stew. Maybe it isn't a *feeling* at all, but rather an unfamiliar building that you wandered into and can't find your way out of. Some of the rooms make you feel afraid, exhausted, hopeless; but every so often, one of them surprises you with a most mysterious joy. By the time you've found the building's exit, you feel a sort of fondness for the time spent inside.

Grief is also irrational. When Dad died in 2008, I spent several weeks believing that the only way I'd ever understand him was to quit college, become an alcoholic myself, and drink until I died. I thought that re-creating his death would give me closure. I can see, now, why that's nonsensical—but at the time, it made complete sense. Still, I miss something about those months of wild grief. I was in such a heightened state that some days it felt like I could reach across the ether and grab Dad's hand. My grief was consuming, drowning out sounds and making my world—because I created my own little spinning planet to mourn in—seem separate from the greater one. I couldn't believe

I ever existed in that *normal* world, where everyone was alive. The death of someone you love splits your timeline in two—before and after. "I'm afraid I will go about for the rest of my life in this one long day, beginning with the day you died," I wrote in my journal on February 22, 2009. As months and years went on and my grief became less acute, I felt farther and farther away from Dad. Eventually, I could go days without thinking of him and I could speak about him without sobbing. I was healthily moving on, but it felt like forgetting.

But grieving *yourself* when you're diagnosed with a chronic illness is different. The emotions might be similar to those felt when mourning a loved one—anger, sadness, numbness, disconnection from reality—but the process of "moving on" is more complicated. Whereas the loss of a loved one has a sense of finality, the loss of self from chronic illness can feel never-ending. Most chronic illnesses work in patterns of flare-ups and remissions, where the disease has an active period and a less active or dormant period, over and over again for a lifetime. I've reached remission twice since my diagnosis, including my current remission, and there was this feeling like, "This is who I am forever now *la dee da dee da!*" I so desperately wished to feel better, long-term, and forget how bad things were at my sickest, despite knowing the unpredictability of my disease and the cruel fact that remission is fleeting. I wanted to pretend, even for a little while, that I was okay again. Denial was sweet but dangerous.

In a 2019 survey of 1,084 people conducted by WebMD and the National Opinion Research Center at the University of Chicago,[1] 24 percent of people who'd experienced serious illness

---

1. "Grief: Beyond the 5 Stages," published online July 11, 2019; accessed February 2, 2020, https://www.webmd.com/special-reports/grief-stages/20190711/grief-beyond-the-5-stages-survey-methodology.

said they were "still intensely grieving" beyond one year when asked how long their most intense grief lasted. (Eighteen percent of people who'd lost a loved one said the same.) In the same survey, people dealing with a serious illness were most likely to indulge in negative behaviors such as abusing drugs or alcohol, eating too much or too little, and maintaining unhealthy relationships. I didn't turn to drugs, alcohol, or food after my diagnosis (though food became confusing and fear-inducing), but I did fall back into a toxic relationship with a boyfriend named Jimmy. Being with Jimmy tethered me to life pre-diagnosis and let me exist in denial, which for me came with a lot of anger. And when I tried to squash the anger, it led to panic—at its worst, that meant panic attacks that caused me to black out. I didn't recognize then that what I was feeling, among other things, was grief. It should have been familiar to me, as death wiped out an entire side of my family in less than a decade. But mourning Dad and his brother and his parents, all of whom died in a seven-year span, had some sort of order. According to the Way Things Work, they were *supposed* to die before me. Even though I lost them too early, the laws of nature weren't broken, and that allowed me to make some sense of a thing that, at its core, will never make sense. But when I got sick and learned there was no cure for my disease, it was *myself* who'd been lost, despite continuing to wake up each day. I was still here, and yet I wasn't. It took a long time to realize I was in mourning.

See, chronically ill people grieve two versions of ourselves: the people we were before we got sick and the future, healthy versions that don't exist (or, at least, look much different from what we'd imagined). There's no guidebook for this kind of ongoing self-loss. No Hallmark card that says, "Sorry you'll never be yourself again." When I found out Dad died my junior year of college, the day before winter break, I spent the next month on Mom's couch wondering if I should go back to Northwestern or just kill myself. But when I got sick, I wasn't overcome with sadness. I was enraged—at everything. I was angry to be stuck in a malfunctioning body, that I had to adjust my life around this *thing* I never asked for while my career suffered because of it, and I was pissed at an unpredictable future without anyone who could understand me. I was so mad all the time that I had to consciously squash the hot, rising ball of rage that lived somewhere between my stomach and my throat just to get through regular human interactions. I thought my pain was more valid than anyone else's because it was *mine*. And getting angry felt *good*, even for a few seconds, until eventually it didn't anymore.

Prior to my diagnosis, I didn't know how to deal with anger. It was an emotion that frightened me. Dad's cause of death was liver failure due to alcohol abuse, but I think a lifetime of toxic anger exacerbated his demise. He was scary because he was angry, and so when grief-laden rage bubbled up inside me, it made me afraid. I didn't know where to put it or how to direct it, so I did what I always did when facing something uncomfortable: I squashed it. I thought about feeling like I thought about hunger: If you ignore it long enough, it'll fade away. But, similar to hunger, if you ignore feeling for too long, it'll kill you. Panic attacks were a furious physical reaction to what I was trying hard to stuff away. The grief was forcing its way out, as much as I tried to fight it, through my trembling hands and pounding heart.

Here's what I wish I had known then:

Control is an illusion.

Paul Chafetz, PhD, is a veteran Dallas-based clinical psychologist who specializes in helping adults through life's most difficult transitions, which includes long-term illness. I've interviewed Dr. Chafetz before for my work at the *New York Times* and *New York Magazine* and found him to be warm, honest, and infectiously optimistic. He told me that letting go of the idea of control is vital to the grieving process—easier said than done for most humans, who are built to relish order and sense rather than chaos. "We go through life with an illusion of safety, guaranteed health, even immortality," he said. "Acquiring a chronic illness pierces this illusion, and this is a loss. Grieving this loss is an integral part of adjusting to the illness. But where is it written that we're guaranteed good health? Assuming that this was promised was an illusion all along. Realism hurts, but it's the more mature choice."

Dr. Chafetz was spot-on. I held on to anger, even when it burned me up inside, because I'd lost control of my body and because I'd assumed good health was my right. This wasn't entirely my fault. There's very little public dialogue about chronic illness—we're brought up to believe sickness either goes away or kills you. But what about that space in between, where it does neither? Six in ten Americans exist within that space, living with at least one chronic condition, yet it's rarely talked about outside of doctor's offices or *hush-hush* support groups. Kathleen Gilbert, PhD, is professor emerita at Indiana University and a veteran grief researcher. She's spent the better part of forty years studying different kinds of loss and has published several papers, books, and studies on everything from husbands who've been widowed to how grieving morphed in the age of the internet. "I once interviewed a rabbi whose son had progeria [a rare genetic condition that speeds up the aging process in children]," Dr. Gilbert said on the phone. "He spoke a lot about grief. Eventually he came to the point of: 'Why *not* me?'" There's this myth that young people don't get seriously ill, but as I mentioned before, the age of diagnosis for autoimmune diseases like mine tends to be under thirty-five, and 80 percent of Americans who live with an autoimmune disease are women. Had I known any of this before I got sick at twenty-three, maybe it would have been easier to cope—or at least get to that point of "why *not* me?"

Letting go of control allowed me to release the undirected rage I was carrying around. I'm still angry—have you seen the world?—but not at myself, nor at passing strangers whose lives I silently judge as better or easier than mine. I'm not even mad that I'm sick. Rather, the powerful, vibrating fury in my belly is directed at the politicians who are itching to take away chronically ill folks' already paltry health care. Insurance CEOs getting rich off our suffering. Employers who won't hire us. Employers who fire us. Infrastructures that aren't designed with us in mind. Doctors who don't believe us. An economic system that sees no value in sick or disabled bodies. When it has a purpose, anger can be righteous. Anger can be fuel.

You are *not* doing it wrong.

You've surely heard this before, but I'll write it here anyway: There's no right or wrong way to grieve. No two people do it the same way. The stages of grief—denial, anger, bargaining, depression, and acceptance—popularized by the psychiatrist and end-of-life researcher Elisabeth Kübler-Ross in the late 1960s, aren't law—and over time, they've fallen out of favor for a more fluid grief model. (One mental health professional I interviewed even said, "No research has ever documented that the [five stages] exist.") My point is: Whatever you feel while grieving is valid, in whatever order, at whatever time. "The Kübler-Ross model articulates a meaningful description of various elements of grief, but many times the stages don't happen in order," Matt Lundquist, LCSW, MSEd, a New York–based therapist and the founder of Tribeca Therapy, said via email. I've interviewed Lundquist twice before about chronic illness and mental health, as well as news cycle–related PTSD; his nondiagnostic, creativity-focused approach to therapy is highly suited for the times we live in. "Some stages are more meaningful than others, harder than others, and some less of a challenge for certain folks. I've also found that the idea of stages of grief connotes a picture that's more peaceful than reality, which often involves a fair amount of yelling and screaming and agony," he said.

"I used to lecture about the grief process of those who'd lost their ability to communicate—in some instances, permanently," Dr. Gilbert said. "A teenager with brain trauma was experiencing aphasia [loss of speech], and being an adolescent and all, he didn't want to be 'weird.' His speech pathologist could tell him that he was making progress and that all his feelings were normal, but what really helped him was hearing from *other patients* that his feelings were normal." Grief makes you feel utterly alone, but it also presents an opportunity to connect with other chronically ill people in meaningful ways through in-person and online support meetings, fundraising events, volunteering, or however else you can (and that you're comfortable with). When you share stories with each other, you'll come to realize that there's no proper way to process the tremendous loss that comes with chronic illness. It's a great relief to recognize you aren't "doing it wrong," even if your feelings are not represented in the popular culture grief model.

Acceptance in particular is misleading as a "final" stage because it indicates some sort of conclusion—but for chronically ill folks, that may never exist. (Keep in mind that the stages of grief are based on *terminal* illness.) Karen Conlon, LCSW, the founder of New York's Cohesive Therapy, a cognitive behavioral therapist who began her therapy career working with IBD patients at Mount Sinai and a specialist in the psychological impact of gut disease, told me this: "Acceptance comes in stages and tiers. You don't go from not accepting to accepting every aspect of living with your disease, and you may not have the same level of acceptance forever." What's more important than total acceptance is *flexibility*, and a willingness to adapt to the needs your illness requires. "I ask patients to think about what they love to do," Conlon said. "Can you accommodate some of that with the changes to your body? Will this be an opportunity to discover a new skill or a new chapter of your life? New likes?" Conlon is right: According to the Anxiety and Depression Association of America, acceptance for people with chronic illness comes from a combination of three things: "Recognizing that something cannot be changed, consciously working to adjust expectations, and actively seeking more satisfaction and meaning in the things you can do."[2]

Rather than searching for big, sweeping acceptance, then feeling like a failure when it doesn't come, chronically ill folks can enact small, empowering steps, such as taking our required medications, learning everything we can about how our diseases work, seeing doctors regularly and being prepared for appointments with a list of questions, advocating for our needs and wants, figuring out which foods make us feel good, and going to therapy and/or connecting with a support group. "Acceptance doesn't mean that you get over it, or that you're even okay with the loss that comes with becoming chronically ill," Claire Bidwell Smith, LCPC, a writer and grief counselor, said on

2 Paul Greene, "Living with Chronic Illness," Anxiety and Depression Association of America, last updated 2019; accessed February 24, 2020, https://adaa.org/learn-from-us/from-the-experts/blog-posts/consumer/living-chronic-illness.

the phone from her home in South Carolina. "It simply means you're learning to live with the idea and knowledge of it, while holding space to grieve."

Though there's no wrong way to grieve, you should still keep an eye out for signs that indicate you need extra help navigating the loss that comes with chronic illness. I think everyone can use professional help while they're grieving, even if they're handling it "well." Mental health care shouldn't be reserved for crises only. But below are the telltale indicators that you need help putting the train back on its tracks.

- You're having trouble doing daily tasks, like bathing and feeding yourself and/or your children.
- You're skipping work often.
- You're sleeping too much or not enough.
- You're eating too much or not enough.
- You're using alcohol or drugs in an attempt to numb your feelings.
- You're isolating.
- You're falling into destructive behaviors.
- You're having thoughts of self-harm or suicide.

If any of these statements ring true, it's time to reach out for help from a mental health professional. There is *no shame* in this. (If you're not sure where to begin, flip to Appendix II, "How to Find a Good Therapist," in the back of the book, as well as Appendix III, "Mental Health Resources.")

Anxiety is part of grief.

If you think about anxiety as your brain trying to distract you from trauma, it makes sense that it would pop up in the wake of chronic illness. After all, being diagnosed with a chronic illness is trauma. Experiencing the symptoms, *the physical pain*, that come along with chronic illness is trauma. Being hospitalized and subjected to invasive procedures is trauma. Not being believed about your illness is trauma. Losing work and any sort of financial anchor due to illness is trauma. Relationships falling out because of your illness is trauma. Losing autonomy or the ability to do things you love is trauma. Your brain doesn't want to unpack all of these traumatic realities because *it hurts*. Anxious thoughts and behaviors serve as a distraction, a protective mechanism of sorts. Worrying or feeling afraid, occasionally or even often, is pretty normal. After all, these feelings are important protective mechanisms and do serve a purpose to alert us to and keep us from harm. "Humans are hardwired to be vigilant for danger—always looking forward and anticipating," Dr. Chafetz said. "'Anxiety'—a word people often use for when they're feeling fear—is anticipating a future event and feeling a strong need to prepare."

But anxiety becomes disordered when you worry excessively for months on end, and that worrying impacts your life, work, and relationships.[3] (For more about anxiety, flip to Appendix IV, "Chronic Illness and Anxiety.") Don't dismiss changes in mind or body as par for the course or a "normal" part of chronic illness—talk to your health-care providers. Whatever's going on, you deserve to feel better. "Your brain is a unique organ, just like your stomach or your heart," Conlon said. "If you're willing to take care of those organs, then why not treat your brain? Our daily function relies on it."

I'd battled anxiety for most of my life—and continue

3. "Anxiety Disorders," National Institute of Mental Health, last updated July 2018; accessed February 11, 2020, https://www.nimh.nih.gov/health/topics /anxiety-disorders/index.shtml.

to—but after my diagnosis and first hospitalization it made itself undeniable through panic attacks. Turns out, I learned through therapy and chronic illness support groups, that a lot of other people experience anxiety as they grieve. Claire Bidwell Smith wrote an entire book about it called *Anxiety: The Missing Stage of Grief.* "There's a multitude of emotions that come with grief. They can come up quickly and that can be scary," she said. "People often tamp those feelings down and that's one of many reasons anxiety pops up."

The solution? Allow yourself to *feel*. Sounds easy, doesn't it? Well, if you're like me, it isn't. Vulnerability wasn't rewarded as I grew up and feelings were not spoken aloud. Dad's emotions were all over the place—more so when he was drunk, which was, eventually, all the time. Sometimes he'd be screaming about the world wronging him, and other times he'd be sobbing over cheese fries about "the light" going out in a hunted deer's eyes (which happened at a Steak 'n Shake when I was fourteen). Turbulent feelings scared me, and I came to think of *all* emotions as unsafe. I put off going to therapy for so long partly because I was afraid to cry during a session. (I did cry. My psychiatrist handed me a box of tissues. The world kept turning.) Allowing myself time and space to *feel*, even for an hour-long therapy session, seemed indulgent at first. But those thoughts subsided as I began to unpack why I felt that way, and as I started to see and feel real progress from therapy and medication.

Chronically ill people spend a lot of time wishing for the past and worrying about the future, but very little brain space is given to the present. "This is part of grief," Lundquist said. "That you thought your world was going to look a certain way and now you not only have to change how you see your life, but also rethink how you go about constructing hope and finding meaning." This is where mindfulness comes in. "Mindfulness" is one of those words that's become so popular in recent years that it's lost some practical value while simultaneously becoming an extremely profitable industry. But for us chronically ill folks, it simply means to be present and aware of the moment we're in, be it through meditation or something else. You don't need to pay for an app or a book or a class unless you want to.

"Mindfulness must be tailored to the individual," Caryl Boehnert, PhD, a longtime clinical psychologist who specializes in chronic illness and chronic pain, told me on the phone from her office in Minnesota. Dr. Boehnert's postdoctoral fellowship in health psychology set her on the path to focusing on acutely and chronically ill patients, which is what she's been doing since the 1980s. "[Mindfulness] can be the standard breathing exercises to manage autonomic responses, but it can also be sketching, examining a photograph and staying still in the moment with that image, or listening to music or other beautiful sounds," she said. I tried the whole eyes-closed-counting-my-breath thing—I even took a class and downloaded several apps—but I never grasped it. Mindfulness for me comes when I'm writing. Sitting alone searching for the right words, putting thoughts and ideas and memories to a page, hearing the clicks of the keys, feeling the *zap* from my brain to my fingers—that's when I feel the most *in* my body.

Mindfulness is whatever ritual grounds you in the present. Even if it's just a moment to take a few deep breaths and thank your chronically ill body for getting you this far, that's mindfulness. "Working through anxiety requires people to come back to the present," Conlon said. "Anxiety is fueled by fear of the unknown or fear from the past—like a medication previously failing or having an accident in public. Understand that that might not happen again in the future. You aren't a fortune teller!"

In therapy, you'll learn and practice many tools to cope with anxiety. Conlon recommended a simple mindfulness-based one called GLAD that I quite liked when I tried it. You can do this mentally or in a journal. Either way, it only takes a few minutes and is an easy trick to separate your brain from an anxiety spiral and refocus it elsewhere. Here's how it works:

G: Gratitude. Think of one thing, no matter how small, that you're thankful for *today* (keep it focused on today). "I'm thankful that my pain level was a three instead of a five," for example. Spend some time in that feeling.

L: Learning. Name one thing you learned today. Again, it doesn't have to be a giant lightbulb moment. "I learned that eight hours of sleep is the right amount for me," or "I learned that raw vegetables increase my abdominal pain." Appreciate your ability to learn new things every day.

A: Reflect on an accomplishment. One thing you accomplished today, like "I took my medication on time" or "I ate foods that don't cause me any pain" or "I discovered a good anxiety-management exercise."

D: Jot down or think about a delight. One thing that pleased you today, like a cute dog in your neighborhood or a delicious cup of coffee. This can be silly, adorable, funny, whatever! Honor the happiness that brought, no matter how brief. Recreate that joyful feeling by playing it again in your mind, noticing how cool it is that we have the ability to recall stuff that makes us feel good.

Guilt is a part of grief, too.

I don't know *anyone* with chronic illness who hasn't struggled with guilt. We all think we could have done something—many things—differently to prevent getting sick in the first place, and then we feel guilty about needing to rest, not working longer hours, being a "bad" parent or partner, losing relationships, skipping social events, needing extra support and care, and on and on. Guilt and anxiety are friends. They both let us go down the *would have should have could have* rabbit hole, which is an easy place to get stuck. "Guilt is the appropriate emotion when we believe we've done something wrong—violated a rule or commandment or when we believe we've been 'bad,'" Dr. Chafetz said. "Then we're ashamed to be a bad person. But in the vast majority of cases, that's just not true. When there's no direct causation between behavior and chronic illness, then [we shouldn't feel] guilt—we can feel regret, sure, or understand that it's just a darn shame."

Dr. Boehnert offered three strategies that chronically ill people can use to deal with this anxiety-guilt spinout. First, identify cognitive distortions (this is a major part of the work done in cognitive behavioral therapy). "We all have errors in thinking that are left over from childhood," Dr. Boehnert said. "Bad forecasting. Catastrophizing. Looking at the future with only grimness. Thinking you could have done something better, that you shouldn't feel tired, that you'll never get over something, that you'll die miserably." Identifying patterns and figuring out why you think about things the way you do can be the first step to changing those thought patterns. To help you organize this process, I recommend buying a CBT workbook and dedicating a bit of time to it every day. (This isn't a replacement for therapy, but it's a good place to start.)

Next, try an exercise called thought blocking. "This is a technique that people can learn to do once they identify the unhelpful things they're telling themselves," Dr. Boehnert said. "For example, most women have told themselves at one point or another that they're fat, ugly, or stupid. We start with counting how many times per day you're using those words. Once you're actively recognizing the word or thought, you can 'block' it by substituting in a healthier, more positive word or thought." Many chronically ill folks believe they're a burden on their loved ones, so this exercise could be useful every time that thought pops up. Change "I'm a burden" to "I have value" or "I am loved," for example. Noticing your internal dialogue *at all* is progress, so give yourself credit for that.

Last, schedule a time to worry. It's unrealistic to tell chronically ill people to stop worrying entirely; after all, a lot of our fears are valid. "If you can't stop worrying, then schedule a time to worry," Dr. Boehnert said. "Say, from 7:00 to 7:30 a.m., that's the *only* time I will allow myself to worry about this thought. A lot of my patients are, despite chronic illness, very high-functioning people who've scheduled the rest of their lives, so why not schedule a worry time? Set an alarm. Once the clock rings, you stop until the next scheduled session." You can incorporate a worry journal into this practice, too, Dr. Boehnert said.

Worrying—if done right—can be constructive for chronically ill people. "It's okay to worry about the future. It's what human beings do," Conlon said. "But you have to focus on things you can control. Shift the focus from worrying to *planning*." For example, yes, it's possible that your medication might fail. You can't control how your body will react, but you can plan for what you'll do if it does fail. Talk to your doctor about what happens if you need to switch treatments. Know which medication you'll try next. Figure out if you need insurance approvals. Be prepared for new side effects. That's *active* planning, not passive worrying.

"I suggest people shift their word choice to *if-then*, so they can take more practical steps," Dr. Chafetz told me. "It's helpful to identify the fearful event and then apply *if-then*." For example: If my medication stops working, then I've discussed the next option with my doctor. If I need surgery, then I'll research everything I can about it and be sure I choose a skilled, trustworthy surgeon. If I'm treated as a drug seeker, then I can have my doctor put a pain contract in my patient file. A pain contract, also called a pain treatment agreement, lays out why, how often, and at what dosage a patient takes opioids; it can be helpful to have on file if you're chronically ill and require frequent or occasional pain management via ER.

Don't try to rush "meaning."

During an interview on *Ellen* in November 2019, the iconic Julie Andrews said that one of the hardest things she'd ever been through was the loss of her singing voice. She'd tied up her entire identity in that voice and when it was fractured (due to throat surgery gone wrong), she felt an immense amount of grief. Her daughter, a writer with whom Andrews has co-authored several books, finally told her, "Mom, when you write, you're still using your voice. You're just using it in a different way." Andrews said that as soon as she heard that, her grief lifted. She wasn't harnessing her voice in the same way, but she was still using it—and that gave her purpose. She found new meaning. That doesn't mean that she's okay with the loss of her ability to sing or that she doesn't miss doing a thing she loves, but she *can* move forward. Andrews said it took her several years to get to that place, even with the help of therapy.

Like acceptance, "meaning" isn't an end zone, and it may change or look differently over time. "You're making meaning throughout the entire grief process," Dr. Gilbert said. "People want it to be meaning with a capital M, but really it's about finding an explanation for what happened that lets you move on with life. For people who are chronically ill, that has to begin with forgiving themselves for not being able to be the person they imagined themselves as."

You're (more than likely) going to need professional help.

I'll repeat this more times than is necessary: Good help exists for folks like us, and there's no shame in seeking it. I'd argue that's it's not only okay to get mental health help when you're chronically ill, it's *required*. "Any therapist worth their salt should be able to help with grief," Lundquist said. "What is therapy but the activity of helping people grieve?"

Most therapy is so expensive that it's reserved for a certain class of people who can afford it, and it's going to remain that way until our entire health-care system gets a necessary overhaul. But we're also living in a golden age of mental health access where you can connect with a therapist in more ways than ever. (Keep in mind, though, that quantity doesn't mean quality. Just because a lot of mental health options are available doesn't mean they're *good* or the right fit for you. It can take time and effort to find the right match.) If you don't have the physical or mental energy to research mental health professionals, ask a trusted friend or family member for help. Reach out to multiple therapists or counselors to find out what their approach toward chronic illness and grief is. Make sure they take your insurance or offer sliding scale payment. Research community-based mental health care through your local hospitals—sometimes it's discounted or free. If you're a student yourself, take advantage of your campus's mental health center; if you aren't a student but live near a campus with a psychology training program, call and ask what reduced-fee services they provide. If you're homebound, some mental health pros will come to you, or you can do video or phone sessions. There are even reasonably priced therapy apps now that connect you with a therapist via text. (Again, you can find more information in Appendices II and III.)

Chronic illness often feels inescapable, and the desire to be free from a body in pain, a body that's lost control, is understandable. I've wished to leave my body many times, even just for a few moments of relief. I get it. If your feelings of loss are overwhelming and you feel suicidal, please don't suffer in silence. Reach out to your therapist, your support group, a friend or family member you trust, or call the National Suicide Prevention Lifeline. The hotline isn't robust mental health care or a substitute for therapy, of course, but it's open twenty-four hours a day, seven days a week at 1-800-273-8255. I called several years ago and a very kind woman listened to me when I needed someone to *just listen*. No judgment. I felt a lot better after that phone call. There's also an online chat available twenty-four hours a day, seven days a week at suicidepreventionlifeline.org. Now read this sentence (and then read it again if you need to): *My life has meaning and is worth living, even if it looks different than I'd hoped.*

There's this grief analogy I think about a lot, which I first read in a tweet by @LaurenHerschel. Grief is like a box with a ball and a "pain button" inside. Every time the ball hits the pain button, it hurts. At first, the ball is so giant that it hits the button all the time and the pain is inescapable. Over time, the ball shrinks. It connects with the pain button less often. But when the now smaller ball hits the button, it still hurts as much as it ever did. Along those lines, Dr. Gilbert told me that grief is akin to a river: sometimes turbulent, sometimes calm, even comforting.

Grieving makes you realize that two feelings—and three feelings, and four feelings—can exist at once. "I had a parent who'd lost a twin in utero; the other was born healthy. She became frustrated when people told her she should be grateful for the living twin," Dr. Gilbert said. "What they didn't understand is that this mother was grateful *and* grieving." Bidwell Smith said something similar: "Finding a meaningful life doesn't mean you have to let go of grief. People feel like they have to pick sadness or joy. But you can continue to feel sad and create a meaningful, joyful life again." Hear that? *You can feel sad and create a meaningful, joyful life. You can feel sad and create a meaningful, joyful life.*

CHAPTER 5

Old Trauma,
New Trauma

I spent my formative years in the rural Midwest, where everyone was nice and polite but thoroughly fucked-up. No one there went to therapy—or if they did, it was with a church leader under the guise of "spiritual guidance." Though everyone in New York seemed to proudly have a therapist, in my first few years in the city, I still thought therapy was frivolous, something reserved for bored, rich people—or worse, for people I'd watched as a kid on trashy after-school talk shows, guests with compulsive disorders or aversions whose "therapists" made them lick dumpsters or get in a tank full of snakes. Circa 2011, I'd sought out a therapist who specialized in body dysmorphic disorder but bailed after two sessions when she started pushing "exposure therapy." (At that time, I couldn't think of anything scarier than looking at myself in a well-lit mirror.) Instead of searching for a therapist better suited to my needs, I'd given up altogether, unaware of how much I'd need help two and a half years later.

In the summer of 2013, as I recovered from *C. diff* and learned how to live with IBD, I scoured Craigslist for a solo apartment.

I wasn't sure if I could afford to live alone, but I didn't want to risk sharing a bathroom or being sick for extended periods in a shared space. I was tired of trudging to the bathroom ten, fifteen, twenty times through a roommate's dinner party, or explaining why I was in bed for the seventeenth day in a row. I didn't want my roommate's normal, young-person life to change because I was sick. They should be able to have people over and play music and be loud and laugh and dance. *I* was the weirdo. I needed to find my own space to be alone, incurable, unfixable. My health had improved thanks to the transplant, but I still had daily IBD symptoms—pain, urgency, fatigue—and the lingering fear of the unknown. I wanted privacy.

I rented a four-hundred-square-foot studio apartment on the top floor of a classic brownstone off Nostrand Avenue for $1,100 a month. It had lovely parquet floors and a faux mantel perfect for positioning above a writing desk. I painted the walls a calm blue-gray and hung Dad's old film posters. The building backed up against a Caribbean bakery, so the smell of Jamaican patties—buttery crusts and rich curried meat—floated in through the windows. A local mosque's call to prayer rang out every dawn while the neighborhood was sleepy and still. I loved that apartment, even if a cunning and uncatchable mouse lived behind the stove and an ice storm caused the ceiling above my bed to cave in.

But while I was physically safe, I was not *well* when I lived there. Living alone allowed me to coddle my worst anxiety-driven behaviors in isolation, like sitting in front of the mirror for hours poking and prodding every pore until my face was swollen and bloody—my brain's attempt at distraction from other stuff, like thinking about my illness and recent hospitalization. Though destroying my skin wasn't helpful in the long run, it kept my mind busy and sidetracked me from dealing with lingering trauma—one of my brain's sloppy magic tricks.

And I began working for Lifehacker from home, which meant I didn't leave the apartment for days. Venturing outside put me on high alert. A car horn or a person brushing past—hard to avoid in Brooklyn—ignited my fight, flight, or freeze response ("freeze" is a third mechanism common in childhood trauma survivors who learned that staying still was a way to tolerate or avoid abuse), leaving me agitated and tired. My mental health nose-dived.

The only person I had any real interaction with was my on-again-off-again boyfriend, Jimmy, who lived within walking distance and came over late nights after his bartending shift. But even then, it was little more than sex and sleep. Our last breakup had not been amicable and all of our friends knew we were toxic for each other, so our relationship thrived unhealthily on sneakiness and secrecy.

Meanwhile, I was fixated on every motion of my guts, every undulation, every bowel movement. It's bizarre to observe each liquid or solid or in-between that comes out of you, to become hyperaware—obsessed, even—with your own poop. And on top of that, I was consumed with wondering what caused me to get IBD. Was it because I starved myself from ages twelve to seventeen? Had unbridled stress made my guts turn on me? Did I take antibiotics one too many times? Could it be punishment for misdeeds? Was it internalized trauma from childhood? After all, adverse childhood experiences (ACEs) increase the likelihood of poor health outcomes.[1] I went over and over the possibilities, all of which were rife with self-blame. I knew the best answer,

---

1. Rhitu Chatterjee, "CDC: Childhood Trauma Is a Public Health Issue and We Can Do More to Prevent It," NPR, last updated November 5, 2019; accessed

according to doctors and researchers, was "some combination of genetics and environment," but that wasn't good enough for me. I fixated on the cause, because if I had caused it, then maybe I could cure it. In a strange way, my self-blame was a form of hope. But I'd hit a breaking point.

I recognize now that I was wrong on all counts about who therapy is for, though mental health care does remain inaccessible for people who could really use it due to the outrageous cost. (To this day, I can't go as often as I'd like because it's so costly. In New York City, where everything is expensive, therapy averages $200 to $300/hour. Many providers make you pay up front, and even if your health insurance will reimburse you for part of the cost, it can take months to see any money. When my psychiatrist went out-of-network, I went from paying $20/session to $275.) My prejudiced assumptions about therapy and what it meant to seek professional mental health help let me drag my feet for longer than I should have. It took panicking to the point of blacking out and falling down to make me think, "Huh, something might be wrong here." It's a great regret that I didn't seek help sooner. Years sooner.

Before my first therapy session, I tried to narrow down what I thought and how I felt before the attacks occurred. My illness and recent hospitalizations were top of mind, as was my fear of the future with Crohn's disease, but I also became preoccupied by my childhood and adolescence, my parents' marriage, and Dad's death. Memories and the emotions attached to them that I'd, consciously or not, buried deep in the vault overwhelmed me. And I kept having this recurring thought: *I*

February 5, 2020, https://www.npr.org/sections/health-shots/2019/11/05/77655 0377/cdc-childhood-trauma-is-a-public-health-issue-and-we-can-do-more -prevent-it.

have wasted so much time doing things "right," being a grown-up before I was ready, worrying about the future, taking care of mean men, defining myself through work, pretending to want Special K for dinner and angel food cake for birthdays, showing up for some dude's crappy band, wearing pants at the beach, wearing T-shirts in the pool, laughing at jokes that weren't funny, agonizing over the curve of my belly and the same two zits. So. Much. Time. And now, *I'm sick.* That thought turned over and over in my brain. I was underwater, looking up toward the surface while fully aware I couldn't hold my breath long enough to reach it. *I'm sick and I will never get that time back.*

Could a recent traumatic experience—chronic illness diagnosis, life-threatening infection, fecal transplant—resurface long-buried pain? A kind, soft-spoken psychiatrist in a congenially beige Midtown office explained that, yes, it was possible. New trauma can bring up old trauma, and when your brain doesn't know what to do with it all, it panics. *Of course* you're having panic attacks, the psychiatrist said. Hot embarrassment rose through my cheeks as I spoke, but I did my best to explain the past and present compulsions: squeezing my muscles in certain patterns before sleep, eating bites of food in even numbers so no one would get lonely in my stomach, focusing on different body parts that I thought needed fixing, my tendency to isolate, and the destructive skin picking. I revealed my history of disordered eating, my parents' own traumas, and Dad's addiction and death.

It feels strange to dump out a life's worth of ache on a total stranger. You expect them to point toward the door and say, "I'm sorry, but you are way too fucked-up for me to help. Please leave." But they just nod, smile, and take notes. Therapy isn't pleasant—at least, not for me. Maybe some people enjoy it. I still hate going a decade into the process, even though I can see and feel my progress. Examining one's multitudes is difficult, lifelong work. Peeling back layer after layer to discover the who and what and how of what makes you *you* is painful. (This isn't to say therapy can't be fun or funny—that's true, too.) What you learn in therapy about yourself and your relationships isn't always nice. That shit hurts! It stings, a lot, and sometimes for a long time. But it's *constructive* pain—the deep, tender kind that comes with growth. Being alive at all is hurty stuff, and I've found that trying to bury that part of humanness only increases suffering. Trauma will always hurt, but we can carry it, nurture it, uncover it; or we can hide it and let it feed.

The overwhelming takeaway from my first therapy session wasn't relief, but guilt. I felt that because my physical health was improving, I shouldn't *need* therapy. That a second chance at life should be enough to remedy my mental illness(es). Other people have it much worse than I do, I thought, so why am I here? *Another white girl with daddy issues and a former eating disorder. What a cliché!* I was self-sabotaging. I didn't want to acknowledge that my chronic illness affected me not just physically but also mentally. And I was afraid to tell my secrets, giving voice to the fresh and faded traumas I'd ignored.

It was uncomfortable, but I kept going back, in part because I wished for the psychiatrist to think I was smart and capable and interesting. I fretted over keeping him *entertained*! (I needed to be the best at everything, even therapy.) But over several more visits, as my defenses softened, my psychiatrist explained how I'd been using anxiety and anxiety-driven behaviors as coping mechanisms since childhood. In a backward kind of way, anxiety diverted my brain from focusing on more painful thoughts, and anxiety-driven behavior (i.e., skin picking) was my attempt at comfort. Children who experience trauma learn to protect ourselves through these types of thoughts and behaviors, until eventually those protective mechanisms don't serve us anymore—but they can be difficult to let go of. My psychiatrist told me to think of it this way: We do what we need to survive. And when we're safe, we must let go of the things we don't have use for anymore. Further, he helped me understand that my childhood had given me a great number of gifts, like resilience, self-reliance, and adaptability. While I felt unequipped to face a lifetime of chronic illness, I was more prepared than I'd given myself credit for.

Over the course of these first sessions, my psychiatrist also explained that I likely had PTSD stemming from my chronic illness diagnosis and recent hospitalizations, as well as complex PTSD, or CPTSD, from a childhood with an alcoholic father and from Dad's death. (CPTSD is a newly recognized kind of post-traumatic stress diagnosis meant to focus on long-term trauma rather than onetime events.) It took several months for me to talk about the sexual assault that happened when I was a teenager. I was scared and ashamed and I didn't know how to say these words out loud: "My stepfather's son tried to rape me while I slept." I tried to minimize it: *At least he passed out. It wasn't "technically" rape. Again, others have had it so much worse.* But when I finally told my psychiatrist, he didn't echo any of this faulty rationality. Instead, he said that he suspected I, like many sexual assault survivors, was dealing with post-traumatic stress.

There's ample data to support my PTSD from the assault. A US National Comorbidity Survey report found that 94 percent of women experience PTSD symptoms—which may include anxiety, feeling jumpy or irritable, flashbacks, nightmares, hypervigilance, insomnia, reckless behavior, avoiding certain people and places, and trouble concentrating—after a sexual assault.[2] My PTSD was further complicated by the fact that Mom and my stepdad maintain a relationship with the man who attacked me, and because I had recently grown to rely on my parents more during hospitalizations and bad flare-ups. (I also choose to keep a relationship with them as I love Mom and want her in my life, illness or otherwise, despite her parental shortcomings.) Though I haven't seen my abuser since the night he assaulted me, a translucent connection to him remains intact, which has only been bolstered by my chronic illness and intermittent reliance on my parents as caregivers.

After several sessions, I decided to try a daily SSRI for anxiety, obsessions and compulsions, and PTSD, as well as a situational benzo to offset the panic attacks. I no longer need the benzodiazepine, but I'll be on the SSRI for the rest of my life and that's okay. Any fear I once held about losing my creativity to antidepressants dissipated after I realized that I actually functioned at a healthier, more productive level when my brain was medicated. And most days, PTSD isn't an issue. I go weeks, months even, without thinking about it, and then a man will pass too closely in the grocery store or I'll catch a scent similar to Aaron's nauseating blend of hair gel and whiskey. My body reacts extremely—heart racing, sweating, shaking, sometimes vomiting—and I remember: "Oh right. PTSD." (PTSD due to medical trauma is another kind of post-traumatic stress common among chronically ill people. I discuss it in Chapter Ten.)

If chronically ill readers come away with one lesson from this

2. Kaitlin A. Chivers-Wilson, "Sexual Assault and Posttraumatic Stress Disorder: A Review of the Biological, Psychological and Sociological Factors and Treatments," *McGill Journal of Medicine* 9, no. 2 (July 2006): 111–18.

book, I hope it's this: Your body and your brain are not two separate entities. They're a partnership. What happens to your body affects your brain, and what happens to your brain affects your body. Taking care of your brain's health should be no less of a priority than taking care of your body. In a past disease-treatment model, human bodies were looked at like machines: If one part was broken, that part could be fixed independently from the rest, and the machine would function "normally" again. But that model has fallen out of favor as we learn more about the connection between mind and body and as we discover more about chronic illness versus acute illness. If you have a chronic illness, find a doctor who affirms this and a therapist who can help you make sense of your own brain-body connections. Some of your mental health support may come in the form of medication; other help can come from talk therapy. (For more information on how to talk to your therapist about medication, flip to Appendix V, "How to Talk About Mental Health Medication.")

Though medication brought me back from the cliff's edge, it was only one part of the puzzle. To get a true handle on my mental health I had to begin the slow, painstaking process of figuring out what made me the way I was and what kind of person I wanted to be—now, with chronic illness—moving forward. For me, coping with PTSD and anxiety will likely be lifelong work, but just as I've learned what my body needs to manage my physical illness, I'm aware of and prepared for what my brain needs, too.

As you've probably picked up on, my childhood home was unpredictable and because of that, I craved control. I shunned anything that made me feel as though I wasn't in power. My family moved six times and to five states by the time I was in sixth grade. At first it was because Dad got restless and because good opportunities in academia were coming his way; he was a talented documentary filmmaker and teacher who made movies about late-1970s Rastafari culture and worked closely with Grenada's Marxist-Leninist prime minister, Maurice Bishop, building the country's public school system. Bishop, Fidel Castro, "Brother Bob" (as he called Bob Marley), these were his idols until the end. Before Kaetlyn was born in '82 (and before Bishop was executed in '83), my parents came back to the States where Dad worked his way up the ladder to deanship, mostly at community colleges and state schools.

But later, we moved because Dad couldn't keep a job. Mom never seemed to have a say. My parents were progressive in a lot of ways, but not in the man-woman dynamics of their marriage where the wife shut up and sacrificed so the husband could excel (and when the husband stopped excelling, he blamed the wife). That's how I understood relationships: men created pain and women silently absorbed it, like photosynthesis.

At the turn of the millennium, in the wake of another job loss and Kaetlyn's own teenage struggle with drugs and alcohol, Mom and Dad moved us to a tiny, rural town in the middle of Illinois closer to extended family. Somehow, Dad convinced Western Illinois University to hire him. The campus was one hundred miles from our new house, so Dad rented a second small house near campus to cut down on commuting. He could drink as much as he wanted to, alone, there—because Dad never drank with other people. Never at bars or parties. Only alone. In the spring of 2001, he didn't show up for work and the cops couldn't locate him. For days, we thought he was dead and waited for the call that his body had been found. But he wasn't dead—he was holed up in a motel. I wrote about his disappearance in my childhood journal, a purple and yellow hardcover embossed with blue butterflies:

March 1, 2001
I have some bad news. Dad is missing. He hasn't been at work
for the past two days, hasn't been at his house, hasn't called,
and his car is gone. I'm afraid he's dead. I don't know what to
do. I am empty in my heart.

Dad didn't keep the job at Western long. Employment tethered him to some sense of reality, but without it, he was in a free fall. If he was awake, he was drinking. He hid beer cans in his TV cabinet and under the bathroom sink. Sometimes he passed out in the bathtub with the door locked while we pounded on the door, worried that he'd drown. We eventually convinced him to enroll in an inpatient treatment center for alcohol use disorder and depression. He lasted a few days before he decided he was smarter than everyone there and demanded we pick him up and bring him home. That same day, Mom had surgery on a melanoma on the bridge of her nose; what we expected to be minimal was an extensive, face-changing procedure with skin grafts and large stitches. Kaetlyn, still just a kid herself, had to shuttle Mom to and from surgery while coordinating how to bust Dad out of rehab.

With Dad unemployed, we could no longer afford the mortgage, utilities, or car payments. Creditors called so frequently that Dad ripped the phones from the walls. He threatened suicide: "When you come home tonight, you'll find my body," he warned Mom. "You better not let Tessa come in the house first." He was increasingly belligerent, taking out his rage on everyone/

everything from Mom to the dog to the dinner plates, which he liked to smash on the back deck. He slapped Mom so hard that I heard her gasp as the wind was knocked out of her, and I begged her not to call 911 because I was just a kid who didn't know any better.

An argument with Kaetlyn ended with her chasing Dad back to his room with a butcher knife. Barely seventeen, she moved in with her older boyfriend soon after. I understood why she left, but I was frightened without her. Kaetlyn is petite but freakishly strong and scared of nothin', so I always thought if Dad pulled some serious shit, she'd be the one to stop him. So long as I was in her immediate orbit, I felt safe. Mom told me to lock my bedroom door at night, as a precaution, and I did as I was told. Years later during a visit to Brooklyn, she told me that she worried then that Dad would murder me to get back at her for being a "bad wife."

Just before my thirteenth birthday in 2001, Mom signed the lease on a $500-a-month apartment that she wasn't sure she could afford and prepared to leave Dad. She told him her plans to live elsewhere, and that only increased his threats and violence. Our house was in foreclosure. The repo man kept attempting to take the cars. Two dozen feral cats lived on our deck.

Mom and I collected a few things at the house as soundlessly as possible so Dad wouldn't know we were there, but he heard us rummaging around and came out of his room, enraged. He chased us to the car and pried my passenger door open, jumped flat across me, and lunged at Mom. Our three bodies tornadoed together in a spinning pile, limbs flying, voices screaming. He ripped the keys from the ignition and threw them across the yard. "Cunt!" he slurred, punched the car, and stumbled back inside. (I looked up the word *cunt* later on because I hadn't heard it before.) I thought he was going to come back with a knife, so I dashed across the yard for the car keys and raced back to the Mitsubishi. We drove, sweaty and trembling, to my aunt's farmhouse. I sat on the front porch with my cousin, shucking corn, while Mom called the police. Dad was arrested. I never saw my parents together again. They never spoke again, either. At thirteen, I became their default mediator, hounding Dad for seventy-five-dollar child support checks and asking Mom to return boxes of family mementos.

In the wake of Mom and Dad's split, I became concerned with two things: my presentation and my grades. I would be thin and clean and smart. I would maintain a perfect GPA and I wouldn't have sex until I got to college. I would be on Homecoming court and high honor roll. I would be so good and so clean and so smart that no one would suspect that some weeks, my kitchen cabinets were empty. Then, I would choose a university in a major city where I would reinvent myself. Control, as always, was the theme into my twenties.

But chronic illness stopped me in my tracks, stripping away any semblance of authority that I had. I'd always felt dominance over my body—to make it smaller, to study it, to punish it—when external circumstances were beyond my grasp. I could rein my body in as needed until I felt calmer, safer. Crohn's disease removed that power. It made the very thing I used to rein in wild and unpredictable. The phone call was coming from inside the house.

I had my first of about a dozen panic attacks in August 2013, four months after the first fecal transplant. My physical health was manageable as I recovered from *C. diff*, but my anxiety was high, relying on a destructive pattern of isolation, obsessive thoughts, and compulsive skin picking. I woke up every day alone in that small Bed-Stuy studio with a racing heart and a fluttering stomach. One August afternoon, as I sat at my desk, my heart began beating so fast and loud that I could hear it in my eardrums and see it through my shirt. My vision blurred and my hands trembled as they rested on the laptop's keyboard. Thinking I needed to splash some cold water on my face, I got up to go to the sink. But my cheeks flushed hot and I felt unsteady as I stepped toward the faucet.

My heart pounded even harder. *Am I having a heart attack?* I tried to take a calming breath—in through the nose, out through the mouth, just how Mom taught me before choir performances and class representative speeches—but drawing air felt sharp and shallow. My sight got kaleidoscopic, like when you press on your eyeballs to "see stars." *Am I dying?* And then, as fast as I stood up, I fell to the floor. I don't know how long I was there—maybe thirty seconds, maybe an hour—but when I came to, I crawled to bed and slept through the rest of the day, through the night, and into the following morning. It was as though the life force had been drained right out of me. Some internet sleuthing led me to believe I'd had a panic attack, and when I finally sought out therapy that fall, my psychiatrist confirmed it.

I still regret that it took several of these *am I dying?* panic attacks to recognize that I needed help. I needed therapy as a kid, really, and I most definitely should have sought it out as soon as I was diagnosed with IBD. Chronic illness is enough to need professional help. But it doesn't exist in a vacuum. Pain thrives alongside other pain. As my editor vividly illustrated during one of our conversations about this book, everyone carries around these heavy buckets. One bucket might be a traumatic childhood, another an abusive relationship, a third the loss of a loved one, a fourth an unfulfilling career. Add to that mix incurable illness, a very full bucket that you must carry for the rest of your life, and it becomes too unwieldy to carry alone. You have to decide which buckets you can set down and which you can lighten. That's where therapy helps.

When Dad died in 2008 during my junior year of college, his death became another heavy bucket. I was relieved, in a way that anyone who's loved an addict will understand, that he was gone, but I still missed him desperately. Dad was confusing because knowing him was like knowing two people: sober Dad and not-sober Dad. If addiction is a disease, which the research supports, then Dad was chronically ill, too. I wish that made the hard stuff—the arrest for physical violence directed at Mom, the emotional terror rained on Kaetlyn, the involvement in men's rights forums, the lying, the stealing—easier to forgive.

Even during periods of sobriety, Dad was often arrogant and mean. He was a genius, no doubt, but he wielded his intelligence as a weapon to make others feel small. He made rude comments about strangers' looks and weight, so from a young age, thinness and beauty were things important to *me* because they were important to *him*. Dad was combative and liked to argue because he'd win; he was smarter and meaner than any opponent.

Still, he could be sweet and even goofy. He bought us a karaoke machine and never said we were annoying, even though we were. He let us do his makeup, badly, and he participated in imaginary tea parties, fashion shows, and dance performances. He had a solution for everything; if he didn't have one, he'd research until he did, presenting a perfectly organized, color-coded, highlighted portfolio. When both family cars broke down in the Columbia River Gorge, on the seventeen-hundred-mile move from Oregon to Iowa, we didn't worry because Dad would know what to do. For holidays, he made intricate handmade astrology charts, photo albums, and personalized playlists. He took thousands of photos of us as children and recorded hundreds of hours of home video, always the documentarian. He wrote lovely, poetic letters. When I get sad about the way things turned out, I try to remember that he loved his children. I know my father loved his children.

Here's something I learned in therapy: I can redefine my memories, traumas, and experiences to work *for me* instead of whiting them out. I don't need reinvention. When I started doing the work of figuring myself out, I actually liked myself—what a *weird* revelation after a life of self-loathing (made even weirder by the fact that a chronic illness diagnosis sparked this self-discovery). And when I began to see my value, I stopped wanting to be someone else, a far-off future self. I claimed all the strange little piled-up bits, even the ones that used to embarrass or hurt me. And it became easier to deal with other challenges, even massive ones like chronic illness, because I can now set down some of those heavy buckets. I'll still carry chronic illness for the rest of my life, but it feels lighter.

CHAPTER 6

Partners

I met Jimmy the fall I moved to New York. In some ways, we couldn't have been more different: Jimmy was reckless and unpredictable; I was careful and tightly wound. But the magnetic pull was obvious: He was kicking a heroin addiction with Suboxone, a medication that blocks the euphoria of opiates; I was reeling from the death of my addict father. I believed I could help Jimmy get better, and Jimmy thought he could help me loosen up. He took me to raves in Bushwick warehouses and introduced me to artists and musicians, while I offered him security and help, both emotional and financial. We knew how to push each other's buttons—I'd call him worthless, he'd call me crazy—and what should have been nothing more than a fling turned into five years plus an engagement.

In February 2015, Jimmy and I were supposed to go to Paris to celebrate our fourth anniversary, or as much of an anniversary as two people can have when they've broken up a dozen times. But when we got to the airport, TSA staff told us Jimmy's passport was too close to its expiration date. We hastily rescheduled the trip for March.

By then, I was really sick. I thought it was a bad IBD flare but, unknown to me at the time, it was also recurrent *C. diff.* (I'd taken broad-spectrum antibiotics for a monthslong sinus infection after trying every other remedy. The antibiotics disrupted the delicate balance of my gut, creating a perfect environment for the infection to recur. Patients who've had *C. diff* once have an increased risk of getting it again.) Like so many nights, the night before we were due to fly to France, I pretended to be asleep when Jimmy got home after a bartending shift. He worked at the bar until two or sometimes four in the morning, then slept until 1:00 p.m. or later only to get up and do it all over again. He was always drunk when he got home. I'd listen from the bedroom as he dropped his keys on the table, ate leftovers, drank a beer or two, and watched TV.

But this night, he skipped that part. He wanted to fight, and I was the only one around to engage with. He started shouting—I don't remember about what. I sat up in bed to face him, but he pushed me back and got on top of me, pinning my arms down. *Another man on top of me when I don't want him to be.* Struggling was pointless—Jimmy had eighty pounds on me and I was weak from illness. But I still tried to wriggle out from under him. He headbutted me, connecting with the top of my cheekbone where it meets the eye socket. He bit down on the round curve of my shoulder. He wouldn't let me up, even though I pleaded and begged and bargained. For hours. He kept yelling, "Is this what you want? Is this what you want?" I got an arm free and tried to grab my phone to call for help. He saw me reaching for it and chucked it across the bedroom.

As he threw the phone, I was able to slip under him, run to the spare bedroom, and lock the door. He banged on the door and screamed until he passed out in the hall. The next morning, we flew to Paris.

"Last night was really, really bad," I said, as we sat at the airport gate.

He nodded but said nothing.

We didn't talk about it again.

I held it together enough during the day, with lots of Imodium, to see the Louvre and the catacombs. I tried not to think about what had happened before we left, but every time I looked at Jimmy across a café table, I replayed him holding me down, his forehead coming down fast—*smack!*—on my face. Still, I posted photos on social media—cheese plates, paintings, the Eiffel Tower, late-winter gardens—like everything was fine and fun and romantic.

According to the World Health Organization, women with disabilities are much more likely to suffer abuse than their able-bodied peers.[1] Emotionally and physically abusive relationships become even more complex when one partner is chronically ill or disabled, as the receiver of the abuse may need their abuser for financial support, health insurance, shelter, caregiving, and more. A 2013 survey conducted by the Verizon Foundation and *MORE Magazine* found that "women who have experienced domestic violence are significantly more likely to be diagnosed with a chronic health condition than those who have not."[2] Seventy percent of the 1,005 women ages twenty-one and older surveyed reported having at least one chronic condition; this

1. "Violence Against Adults and Children with Disabilities," World Health Organization, updated February 2012; accessed February 3, 2020, https://www.who.int/disabilities/violence/en/.

2. "Exploring the Relationship Between Domestic Violence and Chronic Health Conditions," Verizon Foundation and *MORE Magazine*, published November 2013; accessed February 3, 2020, http://www.ncdsv.org/Verizon-More_Exploring-the-Relationship-between-DV-and-Chronic-Health-Conditions-survey-summary_10-2013.pdf.

went up to 81 percent for women who'd experienced domestic violence.

I wonder, were these women chronically ill when they got with their abusers, and stayed because they felt—as I had in an abusive relationship—that no one else would want them? Or did they get sick after the abuse started? Were the symptoms of their conditions exacerbated by the abuse? Did they stay for financial reasons, or because they relied on their partner's insurance? More research must be done on the link between chronic illness and domestic violence—we've barely scratched the surface. Without a better body of research, this lack of knowledge has real-world ramifications. Health-care providers need the training to speak to their patients about domestic violence, and to help them properly should they discover abuse. We must uncouple health insurance from employment and income, making it affordable (read: free at point of service) for everyone, lessening the grip of financial abuse. We need trained responders who are *not* police; cops are notoriously bad at handling domestic violence, and there's a systemic partner abuse problem within our national police force.[3] And we must establish better systems to help victims who are without the support or financial means to leave, then keep them safe when they do leave (the time when they are most at risk). There are *mountains* of work to do.

If you're in an emotionally or physically abusive relationship and need help getting to safety, you are not alone. There are resources available to you. The National Domestic Violence Hotline is available 24/7 in more than two hundred languages

3. Conor Friedersdorf, "Police Have a Much Bigger Domestic-Abuse Problem Than the NFL Does," *Atlantic*, published September 19, 2014; accessed June 20, 2020, https://www.theatlantic.com/national/archive/2014/09/police-officers-who-hit-their-wives-or-girlfriends/380329/.

at 1-800-799-7233, or you can chat with an advocate online through their website, www.thehotline.org (click "Chat Now" to open a separate, private window—it doesn't download anything onto your computer, if that's a concern). The folks who run the hotline help with: coming up with an escape plan that allows you to exit safely, establishing your emergency network (trusted friends and family, for example), setting you up with safety mechanisms until you're able to leave (i.e., sharing your location with a close friend, creating an emergency word that you can text that lets friends or family know to call 911, etc.), getting you medical care, finding local shelters or safe homes, helping you find legal aid, and connecting you with mental health resources.

And while chronic illness and disability put us at higher risk for emotionally and physically abusive relationships than is the case with our able-bodied peers, dating and intimacy pose particular challenges in even healthy, loving relationships. I hear the same fears expressed in my support groups over and over again: "I'm not like I used to be and I'm afraid my partner is no longer in love with me"; "Sex is so painful that I can't do it anymore and I'm scared my partner will cheat on me or leave"; "I fear that my partner thinks I'm just lazy and faking my symptoms"; "I think my partner is still waiting for me to be 'normal' again, but I don't know how to tell them that's never going to happen"; "I worry my spouse regrets marrying me—I was healthy then and I'm not now"; "I think my partner looks at me as a burden"; "I'm in remission now and am afraid for how my partner will react when my symptoms flare up again." These are heavy issues that can benefit from the help of a therapist who's well versed in couples work, as well as chronic illness. (Yes, I'm plugging therapy again—and it won't be the last time! Mental health support is imperative for chronically ill people, individually or in a partnership.) There are so many questions to unpack in relationships affected by chronic illness, like:

What are both partners' biggest fears? Marissa Moore, LMHC, founder of Therapy Brooklyn and a specialist in couples therapy, dedicated part of her career to working with individuals and couples living with HIV, a disease that incorporates not only the stigma of chronic illness but also the deeply entrenched judgments about who suffers from it. Moore said that fear can arise between couples even when a chronic illness is well managed. "The healthy person worries about their partner's health—there's this wondering if the other shoe is going to drop," Moore said via email. "If they rely on and see their partner as healthy again, will they stay that way and what if it changes? A lot of [therapy] work is around 'what if' questions and managing when and how those questions arise." As fears go unspoken, they fester, which is why therapy can be so beneficial: It gives couples a safe space to discuss and work through fears, resentments, and sadness under the guidance of a trained third party.

How much does each person understand about the illness? In therapy, you might uncover that the healthy partner leans on the chronically ill partner to educate them rather than seeking out information on their own. In turn, the ill partner resents being the primary source of information. Does one partner understand more about the requirements of disease management? Or is neither partner well versed in how the illness works? "Psychoeducation—i.e., helping patients better understand how their chronic illnesses behave—is an essential part of therapy," Cohesive Therapy's Karen Conlon said during one of our phone calls. "The expectation is often life pre–chronic illness and they're still trying to return to that." It's vital that both partners recognize that chronic illness is real, even when one doesn't "look sick," and that it will require lifelong management. Some people are not prepared to stick around for a lifetime of illness, and that's something you'll have to reckon with. Sometimes relationships—even marriages—end due to lack of support for and acceptance of chronic illness.

How are you defining your roles within the relationship? Karen Winkler, PhD, MS, RN, is the founder of Chronic Illness Counseling NYC, a psychotherapist, nurse, community health trainer, and a person with chronic illness. Her approach focuses on the psychodynamic (meaning sometimes unconscious yet deeply felt) dimensions of living in a chronically ill body. She told me that how we identify ourselves influences how we identify in our relationships, too: "The disease can become so integrated into who [we] are, and feel like 'me,' fitting tight to the skin—but it can also feel like 'not me,' a part that feels alien or abject. As a therapist, it's helpful for me to identify this with my patients. It can be confusing for a person to recognize and navigate these shifts in what therapists sometimes call 'self-states,' and understand how this affects our relationships."

Figuring out where your illness falls in how you perceive yourself will uncover patterns in your relationship: Does your disease feel like a central part of who you are or not? Are you afraid of what it means for your sense of self to be chronically ill? Are you pushing away your diagnosis because of fear or denial? For example, if you reject your chronic illness diagnosis, your partner might follow your lead and pretend nothing is wrong—even when your illness flares up and you need their help. And the same is true on the opposite side of the spectrum. "The partner who's healthy might find themselves in a caretaker role, and they may feel pressured or burdened by it," Moore explained. "The person being taken care of might welcome the support but also struggle with feeling like a burden. Having space to talk about these roles and define them more fully helps couples, as they begin to see the roles they've taken on as something they can actively choose and shape over time."

Is empathy a focus in the relationship? "Healthy folks can ask themselves: What is it like to live in an able body? Are there blind spots or assumptions because I'm able-bodied and healthy?" Moore said. "[These questions] have the healthy person look at what health has meant to them and how that might be informing how they're experiencing a [partner] who's chronically ill." This too can go the other way: The chronically ill person needs to think about their partner's stress as a caretaker, the fear they feel over a condition worsening or becoming unmanageable, and the helplessness that accompanies being unable to "fix" the sickness. Chronic illness takes up a lot of space in a relationship, so it's important to give the healthy person as much consideration as the sick partner; their needs may be different, but they're no less significant. "[Partners] may feel guilty about asking for their needs and wants—like it's 'too much,' or that they don't deserve to ask for more," Moore said. "But it's important for couples to open up space to give each other permission to ask for what they need, while also giving permission for the person on the other end to say no."

Are you being specific about what you need from each other? Vijayeta Sinh, PhD, is a New York–based psychologist who's been seeing individuals and couples in practice for nearly fifteen years. As the founder of Therapy Couch NYC, Dr. Sinh also specializes in therapy for LGBTQ+ people who are coming out, dealing with discrimination, and navigating stigma and shame. "It's hard for [healthy] partners to know what their [chronically ill partner's] specific needs for assistance are. It's important for [the chronically ill partner] to ask for help even though this can be challenging and means coming to terms with a disability," she said. "Open communication can help healthy partners better understand and be able to problem solve about which areas they might be able to assist with. If possible, check in with your partner at least twice a month to discuss what you're both experiencing and how it's impacting you."

Check-ins are a time to set goals and see how you're both meeting them (i.e., "At our last check-in, we set a goal that you'd cook dinner twice a week so that I can rest, but I ended up making dinner every night. How can we improve planning and preparing for next week?") and where you're succeeding or need to adjust. Having these on the calendar every two weeks allows both partners to stay on top of issues and solve them together rather than letting things go unspoken and turn into resentment.

Are you communicating about your sexual needs, wants, and boundaries? What we need and want when it comes to sex changes all the time, chronic illness or not. You're allowed to change your mind about what feels good for you, mentally and physically, throughout your life. Sexuality is an evolving thing! And chronic illness brings up a whole host of issues: self-esteem can suffer; people may feel desexualized/dehumanized from the hospitalizations and medical treatments; medication might lower sex drive; pain and discomfort could deem certain sex acts impossible to enjoy; surgeries that result in scarring or a medical device like an ostomy bag may cause shame; and flare-ups might make parts of the body more sensitive to pain than usual. Chronic illness challenges how you think about sex—what it is, what feels good, how you communicate—and how you think about yourself as a sexual being.

Jill McDevitt, PhD, is a sexologist, sexuality educator, and sexual wellness coach who has three academic degrees in human sexuality—more than anyone else on earth (!). On the phone from San Diego, Dr. McDevitt said that as a first step, it's vital for chronically ill people to uncover their internal dialogues—for example, are you constantly telling yourself that you're disgusting and undesirable? A sexual relationship that's healthy, fun, and beneficial starts *within you*, so what kind of foundation are you building if you're speaking cruelly to yourself all day? "We don't even listen when we talk to ourselves—we don't listen to the language," Dr. McDevitt said. "It's important just to notice it, to be aware of the words and the voice we use. This is where mindfulness and journaling can help. Then celebrate it: 'Holy crap, you noticed something and that's great!' Positive reinforcement gets you out of the mindset of always picking on yourself."

Sexual self-care—which Dr. McDevitt defines as "a radical way of refusing to prescribe to societal messages"—helps to build this healthy inner foundation. Ask yourself some questions: Where do my ideas about sex come from? How did I feel during my first sexual experiences? How do I feel during sexual experiences now? Do I need help figuring out past or present sexual traumas? What do I enjoy about sex—and what do I not? Can I think of a time I communicated well about my needs and wants during sex, and a time I could have communicated better? What does my ideal sex life look like? Even if you've thought about these questions before, your answers may change in light of chronic illness. And as you work through them, these answers will help to establish your sexual boundaries—meaning the limits that you're comfortable with—plus how to approach them with your partner(s). "Setting boundaries begins with discussing roadblocks. Is there shame involved? Will there be judgment if I

speak up? What's missing and how do I identify it?" Dr. McDevitt said. "Then we start with baby steps. Write a script and practice it. Make yourself one percent vulnerable to the discussion
and see how it goes, then build from there."

Consent plays a crucial part in the discussion about boundaries. I like Planned Parenthood's definition of the word:
"Consent means actively agreeing to be sexual with someone.
Consent lets someone know that sex is wanted. Sexual activity
without consent is rape or sexual assault." They also created
a cute acronym—FRIES—that stands for **Freely Given** (i.e.,
not under the influence of threats, manipulation, or drugs and
alcohol); **Reversible** (you can revoke consent at *any* point, even
if you said yes at first, or if you're mid-intercourse); **Informed**
(you're knowledgeable about what you've agreed to, like how
far you want to go and what type of protection you'll use);
Enthusiastic (you aren't having sex because you feel like you
have to, you're having sex because you *want* to); and **Specific**
(the boundaries are clear, like if you want to kiss but nothing
more).

Talking about consent can feel awkward, sure, and the goal
isn't to make it *not* awkward. The goal is to be willing to face
the uncomfortableness head-on, together. Dr. McDevitt recommended trying a practice session without sex involved to get
familiar with the language. Here are some simple phrases to get
you started (this goes for online, too, not just IRL! Online sexual experiences are a great way for chronically ill and disabled
people to explore and have fun, but they need to be safe, too):

- Do you want to have sex?
- When you say [harder, faster, slower, touch here, etc.], is
  this what you mean?

- Is it okay if I [do this, touch here, speed up, slow down]?
- If I do this, does it make you feel uncomfortable?
- Do you want to do this? Is there something else you'd rather do?
- Are you in any pain? Will you tell me if you are? (Also worth considering: a safe word that lets your partner know to *immediately* stop when you're in pain. Not a few more thrusts and then stop. *Immediately*.)
- Just checking in: Does this feel good for you?
- Do you want to try something else?
- It's very okay if you want to stop. We can try again, or try something else, later!

Becoming comfortable with this kind of language is crucial when dealing with pain or discomfort during sex, which a lot of chronically ill people are. In fact, the American College of Obstetricians and Gynecologists says that three in four people with vaginas experience painful sex at some point[4]—I'd guess this is even higher for those of us with chronic illnesses, especially those that come with chronic pain and those of the reproductive and digestive systems (those organs are kind of mashed in there together and often a disease in one leads to problems in the other). I should also note here that people with penises experience painful sex as well, but at a much lower rate. There's a massive disparity in how painful vaginal sex gets researched and funded versus something like erectile dysfunction, for example.

"Pain during sex is one of the top three sexual health problems I talk to people about," Dr. McDevitt said. "There's a very

4. "When Sex Is Painful," American College of Obstetricians and Gynecologists, last updated 2017; accessed April 24, 2020, https://www.acog.org/patient-resources/faqs/gynecologic-problems/when-sex-is-painful.

patriarchal, heteronormative idea of penis-vagina that really messes people up. I like to ask my patients: Prove that this is the only way to experience sex. When they try to, they have a hard time! Then I work with them on a smorgasbord concept of sexual pleasure and practice." In other words, think of it as discovering a whole bunch of exciting new options rather than a loss. Andrew Gurza, a disability awareness consultant and host of the podcast Disability After Dark, which focuses on sexuality, queerness, and pleasure, agreed. "Penetrative sex is only one aspect of sex," said Gurza, who lives with spastic, quadriplegic cerebral palsy and uses a wheelchair. "For a long time, I couldn't engage in penetrative sex and I can't engage in receptive penetrative sex . . . so I understand the sensuality of exploring parts of each other's bodies that aren't necessarily penetrative."

People often feel "defective" when they're unable to have penetrative sex, and they may chalk it up to a normal part of living with chronic illness or disability and never seek help. Even when they have seen a doctor, "it's all stress" or "you just need to relax" is far too common a response. They may feel as though illness or disability makes them an unsexual being who's unworthy of pleasure, or that they're "selfish" for seeking medical help. Let me get my megaphone: PAIN DOES NOT HAVE TO BE A NORMAL PART OF SEX. YOU DESERVE TO HAVE SEX AS PAIN-FREE AS POSSIBLE. YOU NEED TO SEE A HEALTH-CARE PROVIDER WHO UNDERSTANDS THIS. YOUR CHRONIC ILLNESS DOES NOT RENDER YOU UNFUCKABLE—OKAY? You aren't selfish for wanting sexual pleasure. You don't need to grin and bear it for the sake of your partner. If it's decided that penetrative sex is no longer possible, know that there are other pleasurable options available, and that it's okay to feel sad over what you've lost. "It's important to let people grieve the loss of penetrative sex. Even when they know that other sexual practices exist, they still like the connection of penetrative intercourse," Dr. McDevitt said. "And when that fails them, they must process that loss."

Chronic illness brings with it such trauma that you'd expect to lose more from it than you gain. It seems counterintuitive, then, that being faced with lifelong illness actually gives you opportunities to reevaluate the things that are serving you and those that aren't, romantic relationships being one. Healthy partnerships make life richer and, with chronic illness, serve as a vital source of love and support and pleasure. But if a partnership is no longer working, you're allowed to move on. Ill-health complicates the process, but support and resources are there if you need them. Your life is not only worth living, but it's worth living with people who value and care for you.

CHAPTER 7

Family

Every evening during the trip to Paris in 2015, my abdomen churned and swelled until my insides felt ready to burst. While Jimmy went out drinking and exploring at my encouragement so I could be alone, I got sick. For hours each night, my guts exploded into loud, excruciating diarrhea streaked with ribbons of mucus and blood. The pain made me call out and throw up. Sweat soaked through my clothing. I've read that at a certain point in childbirth, women feel the involuntary, primal urge to strip their clothes off. I did the same. I thought about going to a French emergency room, but if I could make it *one more day, one more day, one more day*, I could get home and back to my regular hospital in Brooklyn. So I held out. When our return plane landed, I took a taxi from JFK to our apartment, packed a hospital bag, and headed directly to Methodist.

The doctors were hopeful, at first, that it was just an IBD flare with no secondary infection. They started me on strong pain medication, steroids to temper the inflammation, Zofran for nausea, and fluids for dehydration. I could *feel* that something was seriously wrong. I needed help—an advocate—and Jimmy wasn't it. Whenever he visited me in the hospital, he was on his way to drunk or already there. So I asked Mom to come to New York and, like each time before, she did right away. She made arrangements to take indefinite time off from her work—administrative work at a school for kids with behavior disorders and/or on the autism spectrum—for a family emergency and headed east, sleeping on an air mattress in our spare room for the next several weeks. I also took time off from the *Daily Beast* and, later, an indefinite leave of absence.

Mom's anxiety was, and sometimes still can be, severe. During fraught periods in the '90s and early '00s, she'd suddenly drop ten or twenty pounds on an already lanky frame, making her clothes hang off her body like a scarecrow. I understood it then as, "Mom has an upset tummy." Still today, even with medication and counseling, she sometimes has to go to the bathroom half a dozen times before she can leave home. "Bad guts run in my family," she's told me since childhood. Mom retired from her administrative job a few years ago and got a Master Gardener certificate. She's always loved plants, I think, because they're less complicated than humans. She's connected to flora in that way people who grew up close to the earth are. Her family lived off the land, and she inherited the ability to communicate with things that grow from the ground—to know what they need, when they need it. Mom copes with her anxiety by retreating into her internal realm—"Mom world," Kaetlyn and I nicknamed it—and revising history to be less painful. She spends a lot of time somewhere far away from reality, in what I've always imagined is an active and colorful brain-place where she can be her true self. I will never be invited to that place or see that version of her, so in a lot of ways, she remains a stranger.

But during my hospital stint in 2015, Mom was the bravest I've ever seen her. She came to the hospital every day and, because she's innately kind, made fast friends with all the doctors, nurses, techs, and janitors. Some nights she pushed chairs together to sleep on, so she didn't have to leave. When she wasn't with me at Methodist, she was walking our dog, doing laundry, and running errands. She brought me packs upon packs of cotton drugstore underwear that I could throw away after wearing, as well as face moisturizer and body lotion to help me feel slightly more human. When the underwear habit became too expensive, we switched to adult diapers. Mom picked the ones that are supposed to look like real underwear; I knew she chose them to make me feel less bad, as if because they had floral patterns on them, I'd forget I was a young woman wearing a diaper. On the rare days I could eat, she snuck in turkey sandwiches and root beer, the only two things that ever sounded good. (I find mayonnaise repulsive, but I wanted it on my sandwiches then—one of the many weird quirks of illness.)

Shortly after Mom arrived, the hospital lab tested my stool for infection. It took a couple of days for the results of the culture to come back. I was sitting up, elevated in the hospital bed, with Mom next to me when a nurse delivered the results.

"You're positive for *C. diff*, sweetie," she said.

Positive for C. diff. The words rattled around my head.

I opened my mouth to reply, "I understand," but instead of language coming out, loud, ragged sobs burst into the quiet room.

Then, I was wailing, my body rocking back and forth. "NONONONONONONONO!"

Mom tried to comfort me while explaining to the nurse why I was reacting in such a way—that I'd had it before, that I had gotten very sick, that it required a fecal transplant, that my worst fear was becoming reality.

"It's going to kill me."

I screamed and sobbed and rocked. My whole life, I considered myself brave: strong enough to survive my childhood home, to leave my hometown, to strike out on my own in New York. But in that moment, when I turned into nothing more than a scared, crying animal, I realized I wasn't brave. I was afraid—aware more than ever that I had lost all control.

It took me a long while to calm down, but when I did, I immediately switched gears, asking about another fecal transplant. My doctors stopped the high-dose IV steroids because those would only fuel the bacterial infection. The *C. diff* infection had to go away before doctors could tackle the IBD flare, which is what the steroids were for in the first place. They started me on IV vancomycin, the same antibiotic that failed the first time I had *C. diff.* I was adamant that antibiotics wouldn't work—they were nothing more than a Band-Aid. Why keep me on medication that won't work when I could skip ahead to a treatment that does? I told every doctor who would listen: *I need a fecal transplant.*

But things were different in 2015 than they were in 2013 when I had *C. diff* the first time. The FDA was regulating fecal transplants more carefully, and many doctors who'd performed them previously halted the procedure or stopped altogether. Under 2015's FDA guidelines, most FMTs could be performed only in a clinical trial setting. Doc called several gastroenterologists who all said the same thing: "We aren't doing transplants right now." No one wanted to step on the FDA's toes.

While I was hospitalized, I wasn't always kind to Mom, even though she was doing the best she could to care and advocate for me. She often bore the brunt of my anger and frustration because she was the person closest to me, physically and emotionally. She was kinder and more forgiving than I deserved. I was downright mean to her more than once (*more than twice*), and then I'd feel horrible for acting so inconsiderately. But I wanted to be cruel to her. I wanted to hurt her—for not better shielding Kaetlyn and me from abuse, for forcing me to grow up too fast, for blaming me when Aaron assaulted me, and for keeping a relationship with my abuser. In hindsight, my anger toward her during my hospitalizations didn't have much to do with my disease at all. Like I said, chronic illness complicates families.

When I got diagnosed with IBD, I was not at all prepared for how my relationships would change. It was challenging to be a friend when I couldn't get out of bed, and equally to be a partner when the pain made me unable to see beyond myself. I struggled to be a good sister as my own circumstances consumed me, and I failed to be a good daughter when illness bubbled up old bitterness. It was hard to be kind to myself—and to everyone around me—when I hated my body and its apparent betrayal. No matter how much you try to explain, people (yourself included, sometimes most of all) expect you to *get better already*—and when you don't, they resent you, even if they don't mean to. When I got sick, all of my relationships changed. Every single one. Some got stronger, more intimate, more honest. And some ended, for better or worse, casualties of an unfair and misunderstood disease.

When you're chronically ill, what happens in your relationships is called *ambiguous loss*. Ambiguous loss is a type of grief that happens when there's no death. Individuals are physically present, but parts of what made them "them" are lost, whether it be, for example, from chronic and/or progressive illness or brain injury. It can also be used when there's no *certain* death, like when a person goes missing or a family member loses contact

with another because of immigration or war. They're not physically around, but they may still feel very much alive in your
mind. Either way, it's defined as having "no certainty that the
person will come back or return to the way they used to be."[1]
According to Dr. Pauline Boss, the therapist and professor who
coined the term, ambiguous loss "confuses families, prevents
resolution of the loss, and freezes the grief process, paralyzing
couple and family functioning." (I would add that this type of
loss affects friendships, too.) For healthy loved ones, you have
to acknowledge that even though your chronically ill friend or
family member is still here, you're grieving parts of them that
have disappeared. And chronically ill people grieve those things
within ourselves, too.

The last decade hasn't been easy for the people I love. It's
understandably heartbreaking to watch someone you care about
get sick and never better. Chronic illness ripples like a stone on a
pond, changing everyone in its waves. There's nothing my loved
ones could have done differently to prevent me from getting
sick, and there's nothing they can do to take it away.

Chronic illness makes parent-child relationships even more
complicated than they already are (which is *very*), whether it's
the parent who's healthy and the child chronically ill, vice versa,
or both—possibly with the same illness, as those sneaky genetics come into play. Guilt is prevalent no matter the dynamic:
healthy and sick parents wonder if they did something to make
their kid sick, healthy kids struggle because their parent is sick
and they aren't, sick kids blame their sick parents for possibly

---

1. "Ambiguous Loss Pioneered by Pauline Boss," University of Minnesota
Department of Family Social Science; accessed March 21, 2020, https://www
.ambiguousloss.com/about/faq/.

passing on an illness or resent (*and then feel guilty for resenting*) that their parents are healthy and they aren't.

"The experience of being diagnosed with chronic illness can be very different developmentally depending on the age at diagnosis. Someone who's diagnosed at, say, age two, is different than a preteen, young adult, or older adult who's lived an entire life without illness," Dr. Karen Winkler told me. "When you're diagnosed at a young age, your parents have to be intimately involved with your body . . . those issues of dependency and autonomy are already loaded, and chronic illness can intensify that." Further: "Children may not even realize the condition is scary, while the parents are terrified about progression, triggers, and emergencies. Or it can go the other way around: the child feels sad and tired and different and the parents are saying, 'You're okay! You're just like everybody else!' Parents may be trying their best to support their child in feeling 'normal,' when to the child, it feels like a very big deal. This can mobilize shame or guilt that can persist into adulthood." Parents must be willing to work with their chronically ill children to set up and test boundaries. How can your kids feel independent while staying safe? How can you give them privacy? This requires open communication and agreed-upon boundaries, like: "I want you to go to the party, but you have to keep your shared location on so I can see where you are"; or, "I need you to text me when you've checked your blood sugar"; or, "I want to send some food with you so that you can be sure it's gluten-free."

For parents, there's a balance between keeping chronically ill kids safe and micromanaging their every move; there's also a fine line between protecting your children and enabling them to never grow into the skills they need as adults. The first step to figuring out this balance? *Talk to your kids.* Ask how you can help them feel safe. Ask how you annoy them. Ask what's working in your parent-kid relationship and what isn't. Ask how they think about their illness, how it fits into their identity. Ask what their day-to-day life with chronic illness is like. Ask about their fears, what they like and don't like about their doctors, and how you can be a better advocate. Let them lead the conversation. When your child is chronically ill, they're your best educational resource on what it's like to live with incurable illness, so utilize that resource.

In addition, joining a support group for parents of chronically ill kids, as well as a support group for adults with your child's diagnosis, would be beneficial; in the former, you can connect over your shared experience as a caregiver, and in the latter, you'll get insight into the unique lives of chronically ill folks. As a parent, you need to see that just because people have the same diagnosis doesn't mean they're destined to the same outcome. Learn as much as you can from a wide variety of people. And look into summer camps for kids with chronic illness (often the counselors have the same diagnosis as the campers), as well as fundraising walks and chronic illness–focused events that the entire family can do together. Bottom line: Make it a priority for your child to feel seen and supported.

One final thing about chronically ill kids: When a child is chronically ill, they may feel confused about body autonomy. Doctors touch them during exams and procedures, parents help them with medical devices, etc. Discussion about consent needs to be front and center between parents and chronically ill children—it's never too early to teach them that they get to decide what happens to their bodies.

Meanwhile, when the parent is chronically ill and the child is healthy, a role reversal can occur, though not always purposefully. "Kids, no matter their developmental age, can struggle with having a chronically ill parent. They grapple with guilt, embarrassment, anger, worry, and fear," Dr. Winkler said. "Who's going to help me? Will I become my parent's caretaker? Will I contract the disease? Will my parent die? Kids want their parents to be invincible. They want to be taken care of, not become the caretaker." Further: "Kids don't want to be different, and having a chronically ill parent can make them feel extremely different. Other kids may ask, 'What's wrong with your mother?' when your mom seems tired or needs a walker or wears an insulin pump." The ill parent might not know how much to share with the child about their illness; they may hide their symptoms and their treatment in an attempt to protect their child, which turns the illness into something scary. Children are incredibly observant, so even if you think you're hiding your illness—you probably aren't. "Kids can benefit from therapy in these situations," Dr. Winkler said. "Individual or family therapy can help kids talk openly about their parent's illness and feel safe expressing their mixed-up emotions of fear, rage, or embarrassment, without feeling their parent will be hurt or retaliate." (You know what else would help parents with chronic illnesses? UNIVERSAL CHILD CARE.)

When kids are little, Dr. Winkler said, it's beneficial to let them feel they're taking an active part in their parent's illness, especially when health crises occur. "[Families can] make charts that document little things like: 'Helped Mom or Dad get out of bed!' Breaking down small steps helps children plot their parent's move to health or recovery and makes them feel more in control and less scared," she added. "They feel helpful rather than [like they're] keeping secrets or being excluded in the face of their parent's illness."

Parents also set the tone in a family when one sibling becomes chronically ill while the other(s) remain healthy. Diane Brennan, LMHC, NCC, is a counselor who specializes in grief in all its forms. As the founder of Life and Loss Mental Health Counseling in New York City, one type of loss she helps patients navigate is sibling loss, however it manifests. "The first step for siblings to work through these complicated emotions is to be aware of them and address them. You need outlets to talk about your feelings and then find ways to work through the losses that are being experienced," Brennan said. "Healthy or ill, you're both experiencing losses, though the emotions relating to those losses are going to be different. It's important to realize there's no right way, wrong way, or singular way to manage those feelings. Find ways to listen to each other, acknowledge the differences, and have compassion for one another." Siblings, as I've been so grateful for with Kaetlyn, turn out to be your best advocates and champions if you can just learn how to talk to each other about difficult stuff.

The greatest gifts a family can give a child are safety and unconditional love. A child cannot be truly safe without unconditional love, and a child is not unconditionally loved if they don't feel safe. Your job as a parent, whether your kid is chronically ill or you are, is to make your relationship a secure, open dialogue. Your kid should know they can come to you with all their questions and fears and jumbled-up emotions, and that in return, you'll listen. You won't respond with anger. Rather, you'll ask questions to better understand, let them vocalize their emotions without shame, and then come up with solutions together. Teach your child empathy by leading with it yourself.

Parents, siblings, partners, and other family members often become caregivers for their chronically ill loved ones; sometimes this work is round-the-clock, or only during active disease periods. (And not all chronically ill people require caregiving—we're capable of living fully independent lives.) Though professional, paid caregivers are involved in some chronically ill people's care, many caregivers are family members who never asked for that role. Indeed, 80 percent of long-term care in the United States is provided by this kind of informal caregiver, 61 percent of whom are women.[2] According to the CDC, the amount of unpaid caregiving by family and friends adds up to $450 million a year.[3] (Chronically ill people are caretakers themselves, too—be it of other ill family members, aging parents, or children with special needs.) It's a stressful, often thankless job that comes with serious effects:

- Between 40 and 70 percent of caregivers report symptoms of depression, including feeling sad or hopeless, eating too much or not enough, sleeping too much or too little, lacking energy, trouble focusing, increasing drug or alcohol use, and thoughts of self-harm.[4]

- Caregiving can bring up other trauma—say you're caring for a parent who was abusive, for example, or you're caring for an ill child while chronically ill yourself—and lead to symptoms of PTSD.

- Caregiving may worsen the caregiver's physical health, including flare-ups of chronic illnesses, fatigue, trouble

2. "Caregiver Issues and Stress," GoodTherapy, last updated November 21, 2019; accessed March 28, 2020, https://www.goodtherapy.org/learn-about -therapy/issues/caregiver-issues.

3. "Caregiving: A Public Health Priority," Centers for Disease Control and Prevention, last updated November 25, 2019; accessed March 28, 2020, https:// www.cdc.gov/aging/caregiving/index.htm.

4. Ibid.

sleeping, headaches, compromised immune systems, and injuries from lifting or moving. And caregivers might put off getting help for themselves, thus worsening the illness or injury and, in turn, making it harder to perform their duties.[5]

- Caregivers experience complicated emotions. While they love the person they're caring for, they may also feel angry, overwhelmed, burned out, resentful, humiliated, isolated, and sad. "Caregivers experience loss related to independence, dreams, privacy, dignity, friendships, work, family life, intellect, and intimacy," Brennan told me. "And, as they're dealing with these things, so is the person they're caring for."

- Twenty-seven percent of caregivers report a moderate to high degree of financial hardships due to caregiving. They may lose paid work and/or put their earned money toward the person they're taking care of.[6]

Support groups are a great outlet for caregivers to connect with others who understand what they're going through. It can be incredibly lonely, and even if you don't want to share at a support meeting, it's beneficial to just gather and listen, or to join a group online. (Note: Support groups make some people feel worse; taking on other folks' trauma can have an adverse effect, leading to greater sadness and overwhelm. In that case, it's not doing you any good.)

And of course, caregivers benefit from individual psychotherapy, too. "[Therapists] can help by commiserating with their

---

5. Ibid.
6. Ibid.

patient and helping them realize that their stress is real and that they're not alone," said Dallas-based Dr. Chafetz, who sees many older couples in caregiver relationships. The process can also help caregivers work through anxiety, fear, resentment, guilt, and all the other complicated feelings that occur hand in hand with love. "Caregivers get support by working with a counselor or therapist individually or in a group," Brennan said. "There are many organizations that offer support and resources to caregivers, too, specifically the Family Caregiver Alliance, National Alliance for Caregiving, and the Rosalynn Carter Institute for Caregiving."

On top of therapy and/or support groups, the Family Caregiver Alliance recommends several strategies to help manage the weight of long-term caregiving, including: hiring professional respite care relief, or asking a trusted friend or family member to look after your loved one, so you can take a break—even short breaks for self-care are restorative; making it a priority to connect with social support; talking to a friend or family member about what you're going through—suffering in silence will only increase the feelings of isolation; not making big decisions for you or your loved one if you're struggling with depression—seek help first; remembering that lifting depression takes time—be kind and patient with yourself.

My relationship with Mom remains complicated. Together, we've been through some of life's most intense challenges, and yet we don't talk about them. Not really. We stick to easy topics like cooking and gardening. And that's okay. I'll be for Mom whatever she needs me to. I don't require an apology from her to carry on or to thrive. Maybe, in her own way, she asks for my forgiveness every time she cares for me, every time she drops everything to rush to my hospital bedside. The older I get, the more I understand that most people—parents included—are doing the best they can with their own heavy buckets. Sometimes Mom's got in the way, sometimes mine did. I forgave her a long time ago.

CHAPTER 8

Ghosts

As March trickled into April 2015, still with no fecal transplant in sight because of the FDA's stringency, I remained adamant that we *had* to find a doctor who'd do the procedure. I would never recover without the FMT. During desperate moments, I read DIY forums and wondered if I could pull off the procedure myself. Professionally, I understood the fear of going up against a powerful government agency. But I was dying. I was twenty-six years old and I was dying, and no one wanted to ruffle feathers to help me *not die*. That was the deepest loneliness I've ever known.

Doc did his best, but he wasn't my in-hospital doctor. An infectious disease doctor, Dr. L., managed my *C. diff* case and we did not get along. I was resolute in asking for a transplant and Dr. L. didn't seem to be doing anything to access one. He kept ordering more antibiotics while I treaded water, testing positive for *C. diff* again and again. He tried several different treatments for the infection, including IV immunoglobulin (IV IG), a treatment for infections and weakened immune systems made from the serum of thousands of blood donors. It caused a bad enough reaction—fever, full-body flushing, nausea, and the feeling that my head was floating away from my body—that a full code team was sent, running, into my room. They stopped the IV IG, injected me with something, and then, *slowwww-lll-yyyy*, my head began to reattach to my shoulders. Mom claimed she saw an angel behind my bed that day: "I asked in prayer if they were there to save you or take you. Save was the answer."

Dr. L. then tried prescribing vancomycin via enema—full IV-style bags of fluid that I was somehow supposed to hold in my pained, diseased rectum and colon. It seemed he was throwing stuff at the wall to see what stuck, yet ignoring my need for a transplant. When I interviewed him for this book, I asked why he wasn't able to access a fecal transplant. He said he "could not recall." There's a lot of bureaucracy in medicine—when multiple doctors handle a patient, they don't want to step on one another's expertise. But Doc kept searching for a specialist to perform a transplant, navigating the delicate balance of in-hospital doctors, overseeing my case, and acting as a mediator between me and the infectious disease doctor, whom I eventually banned from my room unless he was coming in to tell me he'd arranged a transplant.

Weeks passed. I became too weak to walk. My nurses encouraged me to at least shuffle around the room, but I kept falling down. They wrote "FALL RISK" on my dry-erase board. The chance of blood clots goes up when you're bedridden, so I got anticoagulant shots and was hooked up to a compression device that wrapped around my skinny legs, squeezing them over and over again like two giant blood pressure cuffs. Potassium and other electrolytes dripped through my IV, burning like salt in a wound as they traveled up my forearms. Nurses put wide pads, identical to the ones you use to train a puppy, under my butt when I stopped being able to make it to the bathroom. Sometimes, I'd drift off and wake up in my own mess, quick to apologize to the nurses who cleaned me up. "Honey, it's my job," they'd say with a reassuring smile and a pat on my hand. On their next round, they'd bring me ginger candies and giant cups of fresh crushed ice, trying to make me feel better for being a twenty-six-year-old woman who shit the bed. Doctors ordered the medication that kept me alive, but nurses wiped my ass and brought me clean sheets and that kept me *human*. Nurses have this supernatural way, with a knowing look or the squeeze of a hand, to make you think it really is going to be all right.

By May, it was clear that the doctors at Methodist couldn't do anything else for me. Dr. L. transferred me to Columbia, where he thought they could better manage my case, though I felt as if he was giving up. On a late Friday night, an ambulance drove me from Park Slope to Washington Heights. I was flat on a stretcher, watching through the van's back window as streetlights whizzed by above, golden. Mom and Jimmy stayed home to get some rest, though neither of them slept well. Mom had gotten comfortable walking from my apartment near Grand Army Plaza to the hospital in Park Slope, and now she felt a world away from me.

At Columbia, the fluorescent light in my room had a constant flicker that bounced off the yellow walls and made it hard to focus my eyes. There was a foot-wide, crumbling hole in the cinder-block wall where electrical outlets appeared to have once been. The bed moved up and down at the head and foot, over and over again in a pattern, with a loud *whoosh* noise—a pressure bed, the nurse told me, with a broken mechanism. I'd get used to it, she said. I told her I had been on a pain pump, antibiotics, antiemetics, and fluids, among other medications, for several weeks, and could she please start an IV? She'd need the on-call doctor's approval, she said, promising that he would be in soon.

Hours passed. If you've spent much time in hospitals, you know that shifts change on the weekends. Things slow down. Orders take longer. Staff gets short. Finally, a doctor not much older than me came in wearing a mask and carrying a rag. His eyes, the part of his face I could see, were watery and rimmed with red. He apologized for his appearance—a bad head cold—and fired off a list of questions between snorts and sneezes. I got up twice to get sick in the bathroom—as my medication wore off, my symptoms worsened. I asked the doctor to put in an order for vancomycin and Dilaudid, at least, and fluids since I couldn't have anything by mouth (*nil per os*, or NPO, is the medical order). He said he would.

More time passed. When I wasn't sick, I was attempting to rest in an endlessly moving bed. Imagine trying to sleep on a surface that shifts your legs up-up-up, then down-down-down; then your head up-up-up, down-down-down, all while making the sound of air letting out of a semitruck tire. Then, add the initial stages of opiate withdrawal. I couldn't take it any longer. I called Jimmy at 5:30 in the morning.

"You have to get me out of here."

"What? What are you talking about? What's wrong?" He was barely awake.

"The nurse hasn't been here since I got dropped off. I haven't had any medication. I'm getting worse. You have to come pick me up. *Please*."

"Okay. Okay. Let me wake up your mom. We'll be there soon."

"Hurry."

Mom and Jimmy pulled up in a taxi an hour later. Leaving was easy, as I wasn't hooked up to an IV or any machines. As we walked out of the wing, we didn't see a single staff member. "Against Medical Advice," they call it, when a patient leaves without being properly discharged. AMA. But was it AMA if I hadn't received any medical advice in the first place? Even in the best hospitals, patients slip through the cracks.

When we got to our apartment, Mom put a sheet and bed pillow on the couch for me to lie on. She brought me a glass of water, but even the thought of it made me throw up. She tried to spoon the water into my mouth but within seconds of swallowing, I vomited. I could taste every mineral, every speck of dirt, every worm that water had ever come into contact with. Cold, sticky sweat seeped through my clothes, which clung to me like plastic wrap. My bones seemed to be working their way out of my skin, shifting and aching and pushing. I felt a constant, throbbing, uncontrollable need to stretch so I kept flexing my feet against the arm of the couch. Lying on my side, I rocked forward onto my chest and backward onto my shoulder blades, trying to soothe the sensation of my skeleton growing beyond the capacity of my skin. *Pain, everywhere.* Cramps dug mercilessly into my belly. I was suddenly very aware of how many teeth were in my mouth, and it felt like too many. Even the air seemed to have a foul flavor that coated my tongue. The opiates gave everything a fuzzy static, like seeing the world through a smudged lens, but when they wore off abruptly, everything became too bright and too loud and too smelly.

"Please don't let me die," I kept saying. "I don't want to die."

"You just need to hydrate," Mom said, as she tried spooning water into my mouth again. "You'll feel better if you hydrate."

I threw up, again. This went on for hours—Mom spoon-feeding water, me throwing up, Jimmy pacing back and forth. Having gone through heroin withdrawal himself, he recognized what was happening.

"She needs to go back to the hospital," he said, quietly, to Mom. "Now."

Mom and Jimmy called a private ambulance because they feared 911 would take too long—I wasn't in any state to object. (Ten minutes and 0.9 miles to the hospital cost me $3,000.) Paramedics, two guys about my age or younger, hauled me off the couch in a mesh sling and hoisted my frail body onto a stretcher. Back at Methodist, an ER doctor saw the shape I was in.

"Well, you've surely seen better days," he said, standing over me.

I told him as best I could about the IBD flare, *C. diff*, and now, Dilaudid withdrawal. His eyes darted back and forth across my chart, which outlined the weeks I'd been hospitalized there. He looked at my arms and rolled up the bottoms of my leggings to check my legs.

"No veins," he said to one of the nurses standing by. "Go get Boris."

Boris, a surly nurse with a thick Russian accent, gave me a once-over.

"No problem," he said. In what seemed like one swift movement, this stoic ER nurse started an IV in the back of my hand. The familiar smell of isopropyl alcohol filled my nose as the tingly rush of opiates crept up my arm. Thank you, sweet, sweet Boris.

I was then readmitted. Mom asked that I be placed in the

same ward I'd been on before I was sent to Columbia, and I was so relieved to see my familiar nurses. The past forty-eight hours had felt like a surreal dream.

It was around this time that I started to prepare for death. *My life insurance to Zoe. My dog to Mom. My clothes to Kaetlyn for first dibs, then donated. My furniture and books to Jimmy. Would it be uncouth to write my own obituary?* I read about what would happen to my body if I died in the hospital: I'd be transferred to the morgue while my family decided what to do with my refrigerated corpse. Could my organs be donated, or were they too damaged from sickness and medication? Should I bequeath my pathetic body to science? I liked the idea of being buried in that body farm in Texas, where students could study my decomposition.

I now weighed ninety pounds. My skin appeared alien gray and hung from my bones like a saggy, deflated balloon. I relied on someone else for everything: sitting up, putting rubber-bottomed socks on, going to the bathroom, washing up in my room's tiny shower. My body didn't feel like my own. I was ordered not to eat anything but wouldn't have wanted to anyway. Fluids and nutrition came intravenously, though IVs got harder and harder to insert due to all the blown veins. Giant bruises covered my arms in spindly purple and green fireworks next to sore, scabby rashes from all the weeks of medical tape. My veins became so difficult to find that they had to use a machine called a Vein Viewer on my arms, legs, and neck to locate deeper locations less likely to blow up. I left IVs in longer than I should have for fear of not finding another usable spot. (I'm not certain why they didn't insert a port.) My blood pressure was 70/50 on a good day, and some days it wouldn't register at all. The hospital's endocrinologist suspected my adrenal glands were failing; they weren't, I was just sick in lots of other ways. "Were there times you thought I might die?" I asked Mom. "Absolutely," she said.

I knew that I couldn't stay hooked up to IV antibiotics forever but that stopping would free the infection to run rampant. Antibiotics were like a finger in a dam—they tamped things down but weren't a long-term solution. Plus, the IBD flare, which carved my colon and rectum with ulcerations, couldn't be treated safely until the C. diff infection was gone—treatment for IBD required suppressing my immune system, the opposite of what I needed to fight C. diff. Getting better required a fecal transplant first and foremost, but I still couldn't access one.

The only thing that kept me from leaping from a window was the fuzzy euphoria of IV painkillers. Dilaudid, or hydromorphone, is an opioid analgesic that's used for severe pain, like chronic and cancer-related pain. It's chemically similar to morphine but much stronger, earning it the nickname "hospital heroin." During the first few weeks I was admitted, a nurse injected me with 3 milligrams of Dilaudid every four hours (a delivery called IV push); later, the pain management team switched me to a pump for more even and controllable relief. Every thirty minutes I pressed a button to dispense the medication into my forearm. *Click*.

Upon injection, it created a heavy, exploding sensation from the center of my chest outward, like strong hands shoving me backward against the bed. Prickly warmth wove its way through my limbs and up my neck and scalp, followed by a sleepy brain fog that made everything pleasant and dreamlike. Though it didn't always control the physical pain (gastrointestinal pain is notoriously difficult to manage), it made me care less about it. Time passed faster and my anxiety dissipated. I was floating somewhere outside the hospital room in a pink, opiate cloud, and that was *juuuuust* fine. If I slipped into death, at least I wouldn't mind.

Dilaudid has a long list of potential side effects, including sleep disturbances and hallucinations. Though the medication made me tired, I never *really* slept. Opiates disrupt the deeper levels of sleep, including REM, so I wasn't getting any restorative rest. I was somewhere between awake and asleep for weeks at a time. I blame this for Dad, who'd been dead for almost seven years by then, showing up in my hospital room.

Dad died on December 9, 2008. He was fifty-six years old. The coroner thought he'd been dead a few days longer, but that's the day the cops found him. He died on the toilet. For a long time, if I told people he was dead at all, I said he died on the bathroom floor. Like that was somehow more dignified. We cremated him. There was no memorial. The month after he died, I wrote this in my journal:

Dear Dad,

You died December 9th, 2008. Kaetlyn called the police after we couldn't get a hold of you. I knew you were gone when she called me back and all she said was, "Are you home?" I knew then. I was on the sidewalk in the cold when she told me. Her phone rang and it said your name, but when she answered it was not you. It was the coroner.

You were gone.

The world changed in that moment.

The next day, Mom picked me up and took me home. The world looked different. It kept going on without me. And you.

Kaetlyn and I went to the funeral home where your body was.

They told us cremation was a good idea, which means you looked awful. We had to tell them the obituary version of your life.
I think that is all I can handle for now.
You broke my heart.

I love you. Please come back to me.

Please.

In his apartment, there was a meditation mat on the floor and a wooden Buddha statue on the windowsill; an unbuckled wristwatch lay beside the mat. Harold Budd and Brian Eno's *The Pearl*, the same album he played me as a colicky baby, was in the CD player beside his bed. Google searches on his computer included stuff like "LIVER FAILURE BLOATING," "LIVER REGENERATION POSSIBLE," and "WHAT HAPPENS TO BODY DURING CREMATION?" He didn't want to die. In an email several months before his death, he wrote to me: "I will, in all likelihood, live to be 90. When I'm very old, I'd like you and your sister to put me in a rowboat at sunset and push me out to sea."

Kaetlyn and I found other evidence that he'd been sick: used tissues strewn about, a heating pad on the sofa, vomit and feces dried to the carpet as though he couldn't make it to the bathroom in time. No one tells you that when you're poor, you have to clean it up yourself when someone dies. Even your own dad. Kaetlyn and I attempted the cleanup, but seeing Dad's bodily fluids on the floor like that short-circuited our brains. We didn't talk about it and we couldn't fathom going back inside his apartment. Mom and my stepdad took over for us, bagging up Dad's clothes and books. They hired some cheap local cleaners to do the rest—vomit and blood are just that when you don't know who they came from.

A month or so before his death, at Kaetlyn's prompting upon seeing how yellow his skin and eyes had gotten, in addition to his shoddy memory and tendency to repeat things, Dad went to the hospital. He was admitted for liver failure. The doctors told him his liver was 90 percent shot and that he needed a transplant. There was no hope of getting one, though, as alcoholics aren't high on the list. Without a job, Dad didn't have health insurance, so he was afraid of the cost. Plus, he loathed doctors and hospitals. He checked out after a few days. (Sometime after he died, we were notified that the hospital had forgiven his bill. It was dated before his death.) "I almost bit the big one!" he told me on the phone on December 2, the last time I spoke to him. He was scared and swearing a life of sobriety. I sat in my living room on the north side of Chicago, eating ramen noodles, glad that he was out of the hospital but skeptical he'd stay sober. "Well, T.J., I'm rambling," he said. "I'll let you go. I love you." From young childhood, anxiety told me that if I was afraid of it—if I turned fear over and over in my mind until I was sick with worry—that I'd be eventually ready for *that thing*, whatever it was. But I worried about Dad dying for years and I still wasn't prepared to lose him.

When Dad died, I didn't feel his presence or get any messages from beyond like I'd hoped for. But I did see him in a recurring dream: I was in a giant old house—maybe my aunt's farmhouse—running down a staircase with an intricate wood banister. The wall next to the stairs was lined with windows, and I saw Dad's gold Mazda Protégé pull up outside. I rushed to him, screaming, "Where have you been?!" But when I got close, I saw that his eyes—the irises, the whites, everything— were black. That's when I'd wake up.

But in the hospital, high on Dilaudid, my mind had difficulties separating dream from reality. It was nighttime when Dad appeared in my hospital room. The lights were off, though it wasn't dark—the hallway fluorescents shone in constellations through the door, and I kept the TV on for light and comforting background noise. I was in a hazy half-sleep. Dad wore an off-white, short-sleeved shirt, with embroidered brown suns and tortoiseshell buttons. His baseball cap was faded gray with a colorful figure in the center. He stood to the left of the door, calmly, as though he'd always been there. I thought I was dreaming at first—and maybe I was—but my eyes were open. I sat up in bed to look at him. Dad stayed still, his mouth turning upward into a warm smile. His eyes were more blue and clear than they'd been in real life.

Neither of us said anything, but something was communicated: *He knew that I was very sick. I wasn't going to die just yet, but if I did, it was nothing to be afraid of. He would be right here if anything happened.* Then, I blinked, and he wasn't there anymore. I was so sick, so exhausted, and on so much medication that I thought little of it (all I jotted in my hospital notebook was, "Saw Dad tonight") until several months after I'd been discharged. Perhaps it was my brain conjuring a protective mechanism, or the months of Dilaudid and lack of sleep catching up to me. As a journalist it's my job to be skeptical and find a reasonable explanation for phenomena. Maybe "ghosts" are whatever we need them to be, and I needed comfort; Mom's angel was, perhaps, hope. Or maybe ghosts are just grief. Whatever it was, seeing Dad made me less afraid, both in that moment and now, as I face an uncertain future with a disease that can't be cured.

I think of his image in that moment often, happy, in the sun-covered shirt. A version that didn't get to exist on this plane. A best version of him.

"I'll be right here."

CHAPTER 9

Just a Little Longer

Enter Dr. G.

Doc met Dr. G. years prior at a Brooklyn VA hospital where they both worked. Unlike many gastroenterologists, Dr. G. specializes in the treatment of inflammatory bowel disease, particularly in difficult cases like mine. His research focuses on the use of fecal transplants as treatment for *C. diff* and the NOD2 gene that's most prevalent in IBD patients. While I was hospitalized in 2015, Dr. G. took a leadership position in Columbia's IBD program; had he not taken that job and stayed at the VA hospital, I would never have been able to see him. He was new at Columbia, but because of his relationship with Doc, Dr. G. agreed to take me on as a patient and convinced his bosses to allow him to perform the necessary FMT. I was young, I had failed all other treatment, and I wouldn't recover without a transplant. The higher-ups agreed, somewhat begrudgingly, so long as I had a donor who passed a strict approval process. I was thrilled, not just because I'd secured the necessary transplant, but because I truly liked Dr. G., a jovial Irishman with a gleaming smile and a penchant for tailored suits. My bad experience at Columbia didn't dissuade me from pressing ahead with the transplant. I cared about receiving the treatment I desperately needed, not the building I'd receive it in.

The FMT was set up so quickly that there wasn't time to arrange for Zoe to travel to New York, nor did I want to put that burden on her a second time. It's a lot for a kid. Plus, Dr. G. warned that I might need more than one transplant, so my donor should be nearby and available to shit on command. We worked fast to get Jimmy approved as my donor, and after several blood and stool tests, he was. I could stop worrying so much. I'd been through this before and knew how it would go: I'd be asleep for the procedure, which was like a colonoscopy with an added step; then, after I woke up, I'd be uncomfortable as I held in the FMT mixture for as long as possible. For several weeks, my guts would move and rumble as they adjusted to the new bacteria and recovered from the infection. *Easy peasy.*

The only fear I had was that Jimmy's donation wouldn't "work"—that his gut bacteria would somehow be compromised due to his alcohol use. I'd asked him to quit drinking for the sake of his flora (there isn't a ton of research on alcohol's effect on the microbiome, but there's some evidence that it imbalances gut bacteria and leads to inflammation), and to bulk up on "good stuff" in his diet ahead of the transplant—probiotic foods like kimchi and kefir. But he didn't. And I didn't want to lose momentum by starting the donor process over—besides, I didn't know who I'd ask. Columbia wouldn't allow me to use an anonymous donor bank like OpenBiome—the hospital didn't have a relationship with any stool banks then and were skeptical of testing done outside of its own protocols—so I asked the person closest to me. To call on someone for a shit donation requires deep intimacy or total anonymity—anything in between is too weird. It was Jimmy or no one.

I was discharged before the transplant, and I encouraged Mom to return to Illinois. Recovery was on the horizon, I thought, and I wanted her to get back to her normal routine. My doctors agreed to let me taper the antibiotics at home while I waited for the FMT to be scheduled (antibiotic treatment must be stopped for several days before a fecal transplant). I was happy sleeping in my own bed and snuggling my dog, who probably wondered at that point if I'd abandoned him. On transplant day, we took a car from our apartment in Prospect Heights to Columbia's hospital in Washington Heights, carrying Jimmy's turd in a foldable white box that looked like it should have held beautiful pastries instead. Everything started off as expected: I handed off the sample, changed into a gown, got an IV, and smiled at the team that was about to shove liquefied shit into my guts. When no anesthesiologist came to prep me, I figured they were running behind and would be there soon—they tend to be one of the busiest figures in a hospital, running from surgery to surgery and consulting patients and other doctors in between. But Dr. G. arrived, scope in hand, and told me to roll onto my left side—the signal that he was about to start the procedure. People get colonoscopies without anesthesia all the time, but when your guts are torn up *and* you're getting a massive amount of slush transplanted into them, that isn't something you can stand to be awake for.

"Are . . . are you not . . . putting me to sleep?"

Dr. G. said something about not being able to schedule an anesthesiologist in time because they'd organized the transplant so quickly. He inserted the scope. The agony was blinding. The worst of my disease was, and continues to be, in my rectum and lower colon, so the feeling was immediate: white hot, forceful pain and pressure so intense it was as though the scope was ten times its actual circumference. There was no chance it would make its way through my narrow, diseased, infected colon without tearing my insides apart. (Doc, who has done several of my colonoscopies, described my colon like this, verbatim: "You have a tortuous colon, anatomically [note: "tortuous" means I have an abnormally long, loopy colon], and IBD made it worse. Instead of your colon being nicely placed and malleable, it's twisty and turny and scarred. The scope usually moves with me, but your colon is stiff and gives resistance." He went on to compare it to a brick wall. Nice.)

As Dr. G. continued, I clutched the metal sides of the surgical bed with both hands, crying out. The thick smell of the saline and stool mixture caught in my throat and made me gag. I saw my colon on the screens in front of me, alien and angry, as Dr. G. tried to navigate. He commented that it was in worse shape than he anticipated. I knew he'd fought hard to get us here and that I needed the transplant to *not die*, but every centimeter of progress through my diseased large intestine made me gasp. He has to stop, I thought. *He has to stop!*

Just as I was about to scream that I couldn't take it any longer, a charitable nurse injected my IV with Versed, a sedative, and fentanyl, a strong opioid. I remember nothing after that.

For three days following the FMT, I showed signs of improvement. On the fourth day came fever and diarrhea. Seven days later, I tested positive for *C. diff.*

The transplant didn't eradicate the infection, so we had to try again. This time, Dr. G. promised, I'd be asleep from the start. Though I was disappointed that the first transplant didn't work, I was confident the second one would. It had to. I was out of options.

When I woke up from the next transplant, things felt . . . off.

My belly was distended and there was a new kind of swelling sensation throughout my abdomen, as though my colon was rapidly expanding. By nighttime, I was throwing up and feverish. The next day, I was readmitted to Methodist, where doctors ran a series of tests and scans, STAT. They feared I had a bowel perforation or toxic megacolon. Mom frantically flew back to New York. "Since second fecal transplantation, patient never really recovered," Dr. G. wrote in my file. "Ongoing diarrhea, spiking fevers, abdominal pain. Admitted to Methodist Hospital."

Here's what I wrote on June 5, 2015, one week later:

> *Today marks another week in the hospital. I was so angry and confused to end up back here after receiving treatment with an almost perfect success rate. But if I've learned anything these past couple of months, it's that I should expect to be that minuscule percent, that anomaly, that single grain in a stack of rock.*
>
> *Even though I was backed with statistics and hope and the love of an army, the second transplant failed. And it didn't just fail, it made me extremely sick.*
>
> *Basically, the transplant pushed the good E. coli living in my gut (not all E. coli is bad, as long as it stays put and does its job) past the mucosal wall of my large intestine. This is very dangerous.*

As Doc later explained to me, my colon was in such bad shape when I had the fecal transplant that, rather than perforating, something called a "translocation of bacteria" occurred. The *E. coli* from my colon leached into my abdominal cavity, and my immune system was so weak that I ended up with sepsis, an extreme bodily reaction to infection that can result in organ failure and death. Sepsis kills more than a quarter of a million people every year in the United States, according to the CDC.[1]

When doctors discovered the *E. coli* infection, I assumed that I was supposed to die. I'd done all I could to get the fecal transplants, and I thought that would be the turning point. "Just a little longer," I kept telling myself. "Just a little longer," I'd whisper, all those nights in the hospital, when it was hushed and slow. "Hang on just a little longer." I'd been reduced to a single goal: survive. When the transplants didn't go according to plan, I lost my mantra. It had been a little longer and I wasn't any better. If the universe was sending me signs that I wasn't supposed to be here—and not very subtle ones at that—I was reading them loud and clear. Maybe it was time to go.

During the first week of June, a fire sparked by a construction crew started in the basement of Methodist Hospital. Though the fire itself wasn't terribly big and was contained by the FDNY after a couple of hours' work, it produced a massive amount of smoke that traveled through the air ducts and filled multiple floors of the hospital, including mine. We were speedily evacuated. "Can you walk?" a frantic nurse asked me as she ran from room to room figuring out who needed to be carried to safety. I wasn't sure if I could, but I said yes. Shakily, at the pace of someone four times my age, I rolled my IV tower to the designated evacuation point: the maternity ward. New moms with soft postpartum bellies walked the halls slowly, clutching their own IV towers. As I watched them, I prayed for their babies to turn out different than me.

In the days following the fire, thanks to multiple daily

---

1. "Sepsis: Data & Reports," Centers for Disease Control and Prevention, last updated February 14, 2020; accessed March 1, 2020, https://www.cdc.gov/sepsis/datareports/index.html.

antibiotic infusions combined with whatever helpful bacteria that "stuck" from the FMTs, I started to feel better. More good news came from the transplants, too: Based on biopsies and the appearance of the ulceration in my large intestine, my diagnosis was changed to Crohn's disease. I wasn't scared to be diagnosed with Crohn's—I was relieved. I was already living the difficult part: the pain, bleeding, infections, hospitalizations. *That stuff* was scary. Having a name to go along with my symptoms wasn't. A proper diagnosis meant I could begin the right treatment. It gave me hope right as I was preparing to call defeat.

The right diagnosis is a gift not all chronically ill people receive. Many spend years in limbo going from doctor to doctor, test after test, with no certain answers. (Some chronic illnesses don't yet have a diagnostic test. Endometriosis, for example, requires full-on surgery to discover, and understandably, that frightens people from pursuing it.) Too often, sick folks aren't believed about their symptoms, which dissuades them from seeking help. They may self-medicate instead, desperate for relief. Without a diagnosis—and subsequently, without the proper treatment—illnesses get worse. Figuring out what a disease is and giving it a name is often the beginning of less suffering. A step forward.

As I continued to recuperate over the next several days, my blood markers improved, my pain level decreased, and my appetite slowly appeared. Like magic, I started craving turkey sandwiches and root beer.

Doc called it "miraculous."

CHAPTER 10

The Brain and the Self

I was allowed to go home on June 10, 2015. The world was in bloom when I shakily walked out the front doors of Methodist Hospital. Yellow tulips and white flowering trees and green sprouts covered everything like a big, grassy tablecloth—such a contrast to the dull gray winter's end when I was admitted. Flowers don't stop growing just because people go into the hospital. "All of this would be here, even if I wasn't," I thought, and it was oddly calming to feel so small. The next day, June 11, I had my first infusion of infliximab, the immune suppressant biologic medication I'm on to this day.

I equated getting home with being better, but that's another of chronic illness's mean tricks. Some of the most difficult healing happens after you're discharged, outside of the hospital, where your "real" life and your illness overlap and being sick forever becomes confusing, scary, tangible. My body took a long time to heal after months of flaring and infection, even after I began the right medication. My legs were so weak from being bedridden that I fell trying to chase playfully after my dog. I had to sit down in the shower. Jimmy combed my hair and helped me dress. Even cooking a simple meal left me depleted. I was so skinny that

Doc prescribed me high-calorie weight-gain shakes, these chalky fruit-flavored things that came in a juice box. And my eyes were dark and sunken, a fine match to the IV bruises along my arms that faded from purple to green to yellow to gray. Hair fell out in big tufts thanks to the new medication and to telogen effluvium, a phenomenon in which stress or trauma shocks the hair into massive shedding. Pain still radiated through my lower belly and into my rectum. I passed blood and mucus and didn't have a solid bowel movement for weeks after my hospital discharge. Like all New Yorkers, I like things to happen quickly. Waiting for my health to restore was an agonizing lesson in patience.

And while I waited to rebuild my physical strength, I also needed to heal mentally. I was anticipating panic attacks, as those had started after my hospitalizations in 2013, but instead, my brain fluctuated between sleepy numbness and exhausting hypervigilance.

Mental health is unique to every person due to biological, environmental, socioeconomic, and psychological factors, and there's no way we could cover every issue here, so instead I want to briefly discuss two that come up over and over again in my support groups and my conversations with fellow chronically ill folks: depression and PTSD related to medical trauma. (There's more about depression in Appendix VI, "Chronic Illness and Depression"; also check out Appendix VII, "Medical PTSD.")

First, what is depression, really? The word often gets colloquially interchanged for "sadness," and though feeling sad can be part of depression and depression can be sparked by something sad happening, the two aren't the same. "Sadness is not a mental illness," Dr. Paul Chafetz told me. "Sadness is often a completely appropriate emotion. Depression is a much different thing. It's an alteration in brain chemistry—such an alteration that a person cannot feel pleasure." Dr. Chafetz said that the majority of patients he sees aren't clinically depressed—they're grieving a loss of some kind, often a loss of good health. Grief is a perfectly valid reason for seeking mental health help but might not require the same treatment path as depression.

Depression comes with a whole host of symptoms—though you might not experience all of them—that last for two weeks or longer, including:

- Loss of interest in things you once enjoyed
- Weight gain or weight loss; an increase in appetite or feeling little to no interest in food
- Sleeping too much or too little
- Inability to concentrate; feeling like you can't make sense of your work or day-to-day tasks
- Numbness or apathy; you don't feel sad, you just feel nothing
- Feeling worthless
- Lack of energy; feeling fatigued and unmotivated all the time
- Feeling irritable or angry
- An increase in drug or alcohol use
- Thoughts of self-harm or suicide
- Though depression can sometimes look like lethargy, it doesn't always feel like that for the depressed person. It feels like active, inescapable pain.

Depression can cause physical symptoms as well, including body aches, headaches, stomach pain, and other unexplained discomfort. Research shows that depression can increase inflammation, cause changes in heart rate and circulation, and affect the body's stress hormones including an increase in cortisol, which can cause everything from changes in blood pressure and metabolism to acne and memory recall.[1] In other words: Depression can make you feel physically worse, and that isn't helpful at all when you're already ill.

Because symptoms often overlap with those of chronic illness, like changes in appetite or fatigue, depression can be difficult to diagnose. "Many physicians still make the assumption that if you have a chronic illness, then you must be depressed. If you say you're fatigued or appetite suppressed, then they assume depression and prescribe an antidepressant," health psychologist Dr. Caryl Boehnert told me. "But this isn't always the case." On the flip side, chronically ill folks may overlook depression, chalking it up to "normal" symptoms of their physical disease. Further, the medications that treat chronic illness might cause side effects that mimic depression symptoms (like brain fog or fatigue)—or certain medications can even *cause* depression as a side effect. Mental health professionals must do a thorough intake on their chronically ill patients before deciding on treatment, which may or may not include medication, and they should work closely with their patients' other doctors (gastroenterologists, neurologists, etc.) to fully understand how chronic illnesses work and what side effects their current medications may have, as well as potential drug interactions.

Tribeca Therapy's Matt Lundquist explained that diagnosing depression becomes even more complicated for chronically

1. "What Is Cortisol?," Endocrine Society: Hormone Health Network, last updated November 2018, https://www.hormone.org/your-health-and-hormones/glands-and-hormones-a-to-z/hormones/cortisol.

ill people because "diagnostically, depression is thought of as not valid when the [feelings] are an 'appropriate response' to a set of circumstances. That's important because we don't want to pathologize what's called 'ordinary suffering,' or an appropriate emotional response," he said over the phone. "But there's another side of that coin that's significant to those with chronic illness: Depression might be an appropriate response that is, one, nonetheless emotionally distressing and two, not temporary. We need to give attention to those and offer treatment for what may not *technically* qualify diagnostically as depression."

Next, I want to talk about medical PTSD (also called illness-induced PTSD). This kind of post-traumatic stress is criminally under-researched but happens to, according to the body of research that does exist, up to 25 percent of people who go through a life-threatening medical event—that's a whole lot of chronically ill people. It's prevalent in those who've had cancer, experienced a heart attack or stroke, deal with digestive diseases like IBD, patients who've been in an intensive care unit, and people who've given birth. For my fellow IBD-ers, you should know that 41 percent of folks with medical PTSD attribute it to a digestive disease, most commonly Crohn's disease or ulcerative colitis. People with IBD face a 2.4-times increased risk of medical PTSD, according to the National Epidemiologic Survey on Alcohol and Related Conditions, a survey of 36,309 American adults.[2] It's also common in patients who were treated badly or not believed during a medical event.

In "regular" PTSD, triggers are usually external. Treatment

2. Bruce Jancin, "Illness-Induced PTSD Is Common, Understudied," *Clinical Psychiatry News*, last updated May 17, 2017; accessed April 27, 2020, https://www.mdedge.com/psychiatry/article/138435/depression/illness-induced-ptsd-common-understudied.

like talk therapy will help the sufferer understand that they're safe now and that the PTSD-causing event or events are in the past. But medical PTSD is more complicated because the triggers often come from within the patient's body—heart palpitations in a heart attack survivor, for example, or abdominal pain in an IBD patient. Learning how to cope with these internal, somatic triggers—which, in some people, might last a lifetime—is more difficult. According to a report published in the journal *Health Psychology*, "events that pose physical harm or death can shatter one's schemas [note: in psychology, a schema is a deeply engrained way of thinking that helps us organize the world] of a just, purposeful world and an invulnerable self." Dr. Chafetz echoed this: "A life-threatening event is going to sear into your memory and emotions. We're wired that way."

It's not all doom and gloom, though. There's plenty of research that shows how therapy—and even just the sharing of feelings instead of the suppression of them—helps folks with chronic illnesses. For example, in a nine-month randomized study of rheumatoid arthritis patients, one group received individual and group Internal Family Systems (IFS) therapy, a type of psychotherapy that breaks the brain down into three "subpersonalities," each with a different viewpoint; the three subpersonalities are called the exile, the manager, and the firefighter. The other group received information about RA via phone and mail. In the therapy group, the researchers reported that, at the start of the study, when "asked how they were feeling, [participants] almost always replied, 'I'm fine.' Their stoic parts clearly helped them cope, but these managers also kept them in a state of denial. Some shut out their bodily sensations and emotions to the extent that they could not collaborate effectively with their doctors." But at the end of nine months, "the IFS group showed

measurable improvements in their self-assessed joint pain, physical function, self-compassion, and overall pain relative to the
education group. They also showed significant improvements in
depression and self-efficacy."[3]

Further, researchers at the University of Texas at Austin
divided a two-hundred-person psychology class into three groups:
The first group wrote about what was going on in their lives,
the second wrote about the details of a traumatic event, and the
third wrote about a traumatic event as well as the emotions surrounding the event and the impact it had on their lives. The
researchers also asked the class for their health histories. What
they found was this: The third group had a 50 percent drop in
doctor visits compared to the other two groups. "Writing about
their deepest thoughts and feelings about traumas had improved
their mood and resulted in a more optimistic attitude and better physical health," the researchers said. In a follow-up study
of seventy-two students, the researchers recorded as students
spoke about their most traumatic or stressful experience, while a
control group was asked to speak about their plans for the day.
While speaking about trauma or stress, students' blood pressure,
heart rate, and other autonomic functions increased but, after
they'd finished, fell to rates *lower* than before they'd started.
And this drop was still present during six-week follow-ups.[4]
(Have I convinced you yet that burying your feelings isn't doing
you any good? Remember, there's an appendix in the back of the
book that will help you find a therapist.)

Chronic illness also presents an opportunity for what's called
post-traumatic growth. *Post-traumatic growth*, a term coined by

3. Bessel van der Kolk, *The Body Keeps the Score: Brain, Mind, and Body in the Healing of Trauma* (New York: Viking, 2014), 293–94.
4. Ibid., 242.

researchers at the University of North Carolina at Charlotte, is defined as "positive psychological change experienced as a result of adversity and other challenges in order to rise to a higher level of functioning." This kind of growth causes shifts in how we think about ourselves, others, and the world. It forces us to adapt to changes and become less rigid in our thinking. Examples of post-traumatic growth include: a greater appreciation for life, new priorities or a changing order of priorities, more intimate and honest relationships, a new sense of resilience or bravery, recognizing new paths in life or feeling excited by undiscovered options, and a new or rediscovered spiritual or religious practice. Dr. Chafetz added a few more during our phone conversation: learning and being curious, helping others, exploring creative outlets, defining your values and goals, discovering humility, and appreciating something bigger than yourself—be it nature, God, the interconnectedness of people, or the unknown.

After I was discharged from the hospital in 2015, PTSD due to medical trauma showed up for me as insomnia, hyper-vigilance, heightened anxiety, mood swings, and replaying moments where I thought I might die. Several months after I went home that June, I walked past Methodist on my way to Barnes and Noble. I was feeling pretty okay. But as I passed the hospital's doors, sliding open and closed as people went in and out, I abruptly vomited all over the sidewalk. A nurse on a smoke break rushed over. "Are you all right, miss?" I apologized profusely and thanked him, hurrying off embarrassed.

My mental symptoms weren't always so dramatic. But I was irritable and afraid more often than not, which in turn made me feel guilty—just as I'd been in 2013. I'd survived, *again*, and I felt like this, *again*. But this time, I was kinder to myself. I worked through my feelings in therapy and went on a benzodiazepine temporarily to curb panic attacks and poor coping mechanisms. This time around, I had a better understanding of the connection between body and mind, so I worked at healing both. Some sleepless nights, with my palm placed over the steady rhythm of my heart, I was amazed at my body's fragility and its resilience. How could it survive so much yet nearly succumb to something invisible to the naked eye? I may never love my body fully—I am an American woman, after all—but what happened in 2015 made me, for maybe the first time, appreciate this remarkable thing that carries me around. *Look how far we've come.*

Remembering my weeks and months in the hospital now is like imagining a frigid winter day in the oppressive heat of high summer. I've experienced the cold a thousand times, but it's dulled now. Far away. I can describe it, but I can't really *feel* it. And though I'm glad to be home and in stable health, I sometimes miss being in the hospital. I was always trying to get out when I was in, but often when I can't sleep, I imagine the soft clicks and beeps of the IV machine, the glow of the hallway lights, the warm painkiller buzz. It was nice, in a way, to just lie there and be taken care of. To be sick, openly, without worrying about pretending otherwise.

More than any other relationship, the one you harbor with yourself changes most when you're chronically ill. And it's often toxic. Unlike a bad friendship, you're stuck with you— even when you spew the most venomous shit in your internal dialogue. *Worthless, disgusting, unlovable, hopeless, a waste of space, ugly, dumb.* I've called myself all those things and worse. I got stuck in patterns of "should" thinking, going over what I should and shouldn't have done before I got sick, and what I should and shouldn't be doing now that I was sick: I *should* have been [smarter, thinner, nicer, funnier, more opinionated, less opinionated, more charming, less awkward]; I *shouldn't* have [gotten back together with Jimmy, taken time off work, disclosed my illness, *not* disclosed my illness, read so much about my disease online, eaten the "wrong" thing, stressed myself out]. I beat myself up for every single decision, spinning my wheels over what my past and future selves should do differently.

I was being unjustly hard on myself, and that made my brain a horrid place to spend time. "If this was your best friend or a family member and they were having a hard time, what would you say to them? What words would you use? Can you turn that lens of empathy on yourself?" Cohesive Therapy's Karen Conlon asked, going on to explain, "'Should' keeps us stuck. It keeps us feeling guilty and ashamed, like we don't have self-discipline, like we're out of control, like we're deficient. I'm not saying 'should' doesn't have a place in our vocabulary, but you need to be careful in how you're using it and you need to explore what's driving those statements." For chronically ill people, "should" is too often a harmful attempt at regaining the control we sense was lost to illness.

The first step to pushing back on these thoughts is forgiveness. "We, as a species, are really good at stories with beginnings, middles, and ends. In American culture this is especially true," Dr. Kathleen Gilbert, the grief researcher introduced in Chapter Four, told me. "It's one of independence, competence, and 'can do' spirit. Because of this, people think you should be able to overcome anything. But for people who are chronically ill within this culture, they must forgive themselves for not being the person they imagined themselves as."

After forgiveness comes the second step: patience. As much as I wanted to be "cured" of my hostile internal dialogue, that wasn't going to happen overnight. Aiming for my poor self-talk to go away completely wasn't realistic; instead, my goal had to be gradual progress. I had to focus less on the ways I was reacting to my pain and more on the reasons for the pain, because if I didn't uncover the source, I was going to keep running in place. That was—and is—slow work.

From there, I learned to embrace kindness. I'm constantly overriding my initial thoughts about myself—thoughts that are judgmental and harsh—with gentler ones. Humans have the incredible ability to edit ourselves, to replace our learned thoughts and behaviors with relearned ones. Eventually, the relearned thought becomes the natural one—or that's the goal, anyway. Some take longer than others.

But this all leads me to the fourth step: practice. Chronic illness presents an opportunity to reevaluate how you want to address and treat yourself for the rest of your life. Do you want to spend your days convincing yourself that you're repulsive and useless, or do you choose a different internal dialogue? Do you want to make your head a kind, nurturing place to spend time? When you're chronically ill, you can't control how the rest of the world treats you—people will hurt you and let you down and act as though you're less than because of your illness. But your brain doesn't have to echo those individuals. Keep overriding your initial thought with a kinder one. Keep practicing.

Platitudes are annoying, but I've learned over the last decade that sometimes they're true: There *is* light at the end of the tunnel, time *does* heal, and the sun *will* come out tomorrow—so long as you do the work. I didn't figure this out alone and I didn't figure it out overnight. I've spent a lot of time in therapy, a lot of time in support groups, a lot of time finding the right medications, and a lot more time in introspection—and I'm not done. I'm still learning, still healing, still figuring out how my body and my brain work together and separately. This will be a lifelong practice for me, one that takes diligence and seeing myself through a kinder lens than comes naturally.

Some days are still difficult. I want to scream and shake my fists at the world and curse my body. I cry. Some days, I feel *everything*—or even scarier to me, nothing at all. When I have a bunch of these days in a row, I begin to feel as though I live at the bottom of a well with no way out. But then: A bit of rope. Then more. Then enough to grab. As I climb, even slowly, even when I want to let the rope slip because it would be easier than the pain of climbing, I begin to see more and more light. "This work happens slowly," Dr. Chafetz told me. "Understand that there are millions of people who've completed this transition in their minds to being okay with being different, health-wise. Life goes on. The rest of you is still alive, still there. [Chronic illness] forces us to expand our view of what's normal and okay in life. It's growth."

CHAPTER 11

Fight or Flight

When I met Jimmy in late 2010, I was barely twenty-two and he was on the cusp of twenty-three. We met through work—me, an intern at Condé Nast and him, an employee at a company pop-up shop. He shaved his head but always covered it with a beanie and wore layers of mismatched tops and acid-washed jeans with elastic ankles. His thumbnails were painted sky blue and his long, skinny arms were covered in tattoos. I thought he had the face of an angel, or a beautiful alien: pale skin, puffy lips, eyes set above dark bags, gapped teeth. He moved like a shaky dancer, graceful but unsure. His mind always seemed elsewhere. Sometimes when we spoke, I noticed him trembling. When he missed a couple of weeks of work, he told me it was a "bad flu."

Something was weird about him, and the people I worked with talked about it. But I liked him. I liked weird. When he asked for my number, I gave it readily, even though my long-distance college boyfriend and I hadn't *technically* broken up. Months passed. Then, late one February night, a text: "This is Jimmy. I've been away for the last couple months but I'm back in New York now. Do you want to meet for a drink?" I'd never really dated before— I'd had the same boyfriend since the summer before college and by then we'd ended things. Being asked to meet for a drink was exciting. "Can you do tonight?" I replied.

We met up at the unfortunately named Lolita, a bar on the corner of Broome and Allen. It had a neon pink sign and plenty of dark corners. Jimmy looked healthy. He wasn't wearing a hat this time, so I saw that his hair was growing out. The circles under his eyes were lighter. He had on a loose-fitting gray button-down with several buttons undone to show off his smooth, pale chest. Around his neck was a long chain with charms that looked like ancient crests. He was *so cool*, but not effortlessly. He calculated every item of clothing, every tattoo, every text message, every body movement. *Cool* above all else.

We drank and talked and stepped outside to share Parliament Lights, our winter breath mixing with the plumes of cigarette smoke. His uncle had just died, so he had gone home to deliver the eulogy, he told me. He'd studied design at a college on the West Coast but had dropped out short of graduating to move to New York. He played in a bunch of bands that never went anywhere. He liked Graham Greene and Cormac McCarthy. He lived in a loft in Brooklyn, all plywood and milk crates. His parents had recently divorced due to infidelity; Jimmy pretended it didn't bother him but would quietly cry about it after a few drinks.

"People must tell you you're beautiful all the time, huh?" he asked, looking at me closely under pink neon.

We walked back to my apartment on Ludlow and almost immediately had sex. Jimmy was the second person I'd ever slept with. Because he was so drunk, it took him forever to finish. I made the mistake of thinking it was good because it lasted, even if I didn't come and it left me with pain between my legs for two days.

I liked Jimmy less the next morning. He had a certain

charisma when we were drunk, but sober, he was cloying. I didn't know how to ask him to leave. He spent the rest of the day in my tiny room reading books, napping, and trying to press his body into mine. I told him I had work to do and, finally, he left. Minutes later, he texted me a photo of the sunset from the Williamsburg Bridge. Even if he was grating, something about him intrigued me.

On Valentine's Day, another text appeared: "I'd be the luckiest Irish bastard in New York City if you let me take you out tonight." Hours later, he showed up at my door with a dozen bodega roses, and sitting at the waterfront outside the Jane Hotel that night, he told me about his heroin addiction. Somewhere, a small voice within me said, "Save him. Save him like you couldn't save Dad."

Jimmy replaced heroin with alcohol. He drank every single day of our five-year on-again-off-again relationship, with the exception of one thirty-day period spent "drying out." He was deeply insecure without alcohol but never stayed sober long enough to confront his insecurities. A certain amount of booze allowed Jimmy to function, though he rarely stopped there. The more he drank, the angrier he became—always looking for an argument, always violent, always talking shit but never taking responsibility.

Once we started dating, the emotional abuse began right away. First, Jimmy dismissed my concerns about his drinking and consequent behavior; I was "overreacting," "didn't know what I was talking about," or, the harshest, "crazy." He insisted things happened differently than I saw them. My accomplishments were never celebrated; rather, they were an attack on his masculinity. Toward the beginning, when I was certain I wanted nothing more to do with him, he showed up crying on my apartment stoop and wouldn't leave. On and on it went.

Had I not grown up with an addict parent, perhaps I would have ended things sooner. But a lot of Jimmy's behavior was *normal* to me. Dad used similar abuse tactics. It was ordinary. Even now, shamefully, I sometimes remember my relationship with Jimmy as exciting instead of abusive. He was like a black hole—mysterious and beautiful, yet destructive if you got too close.

Jimmy headbutted a guy for speaking to me in a bar. A fight with a taxi driver over an imagined slight spilled out of the car onto a street corner. He destroyed property at his rental building then ducked the bill. Rambling for hours, he tried to convince his visiting cousin to run cocaine across the Mexican border with him—everyone at the table was so confused and secondhand embarrassed that they made excuses to leave. He yelled at me for saying, "I've heard so much about you!" when he introduced me to an acquaintance of his, an up-and-coming musician; Jimmy didn't want her to know he admired her. (*Cool*, remember.) A couple of years into our relationship, when I had to go to the ER for flare-ups, he'd show up late and intoxicated; I sent him home because I was afraid I'd get worse care with him present, or worse, that he'd fight with the staff. We broke up more times than I can count, but it never seemed to stick.

In 2014, we moved into a lovely two-bedroom near Prospect Park. We fought a lot, and I wasn't kind. I found myself scared of him, the same way I was scared of Dad, so making him feel worthless was how I convinced myself that I still had power in our relationship. It was much easier to hurt Jimmy than to help him. Yet, at the same time, I begged him to go to therapy—I'll pay for it. Go back to school and finish your degree—I'll pay for it.

"Why do I need to talk to a therapist when I have you?" he asked.

I set my mind to leave dozens of times, but he'd cry and threaten to self-destruct without me. It was sick, but seeing him beg made me believe I held worth. So I stayed. There's this idea in psychology called "trauma bonding," where people continue bad relationships because they mistake abuse for love. It's often learned in childhood via your caretakers. Trauma-bonded relationships tend to have a fixer and a fixee. The fixer buries their own needs to help or save the fixee, because it's easier to focus on someone else than to care for yourself and your own issues. This kind of bonding creates a multifaceted connection that's difficult to break because trauma bonding can feel *electric*.

Not everything was bad with Jimmy—but it never is in an abusive relationship. That's what keeps you hooked. We had picnics in Prospect Park where we'd spread a pink, worn tapestry under the trees and lie there for hours watching the clouds. We went to concerts and danced until our clothes were damp with sweat. (Jimmy was a fantastic dancer.) We kissed on Lower East Side street corners while people in passing cars honked, yelling, "That is such a New York moment!" He nicknamed me "the duchess" and got a massive thigh tattoo of a crown in my honor. We adopted a dog at the end of 2014 and another during the summer of 2015. We had evenings at home eating pasta and watching *Boardwalk Empire*. It would have been almost normal, if Jimmy didn't need to drink a six-pack to get through dinner. Then he'd go to the bar behind our apartment for more. When I left for the *Daily Beast* office in the mornings, Jimmy would still be asleep. His warm breath smelled like fruit, sweetly rotting.

That night before we left for Paris—when Jimmy pinned me

down, bit me, headbutted me—got shuffled away in its after-
math. I kept the memory a secret, even from myself, because I
believed it was my fault. *I should have left earlier. It's too late to
leave—this is my life now. I must have done something to set him
off. I let Dad die, and I deserve everything bad that happens to me.
I'm sick now and no one else will want me.* I was hospitalized so
soon after it happened that I pushed it out of my mind. Thinking about it wasn't going to help me get better. (Though some
late nights in the hospital, half asleep, I would fantasize about
how I'd kill Jimmy if he ever hit me again.)

Things became even more complicated between us once I
needed Jimmy to be my transplant donor. *Cool guys* don't scoop
up their own poop so that it can be put inside their girlfriend's
butt, but Jimmy went through with it all. I was grateful, but I
think I blamed him, some, when the transplants didn't go exactly
to plan. And I hated feeling indebted to him, as though I needed
to stay regardless of the abuse because he'd done something to
save my life. Looking back now, it's almost like I *couldn't* get
well when I was with Jimmy. I was always worrying about what
would come next, and that fear never let my belly heal.

After the transplants, Jimmy and I had been through something that bonded us through more than shared microbiota. I
thought the emotional and physical abuse would stop then. I'd
almost died. And maybe that powerful experience did bond us
more deeply, for a while. He asked me to marry him with a ring
I bought—a Victorian-era diamond and opal, fittingly shaped
like a teardrop. I don't think we even wanted to be married, but
it felt like what you do after one partner almost kicks the bucket.
We played along and chose a date (October 9), venue (Prospect
Park Boathouse), suit (navy), dress (ivory lace), flowers (antique
roses), food (chicken), invitations (Art Deco). I was convinced if

I planned the perfect wedding everyone would believe I had the perfect relationship. And then, maybe, I'd think it, too.

During the spring of 2016, Jimmy lost weight and started locking the door while he showered. We had a silly birthday party for our second dog, and he nodded out on the couch surrounded by people and loud music. I knew something was wrong, and though it's a breach of trust, I went through his text messages while he slept.

"Hey man, can you bring me more pills? This is the last time, I promise."

I confronted him about it. The pills were for his friend Larry, he said. I could even call Larry to ask. I did. Larry said the pills were indeed for him and he was sorry for any confusion.

A week or so later, I found white, round pain pills in Jimmy's coat pocket. "They must be left over from when I got them for Larry," he said. "Flush them if you want to." So calm. So *cool*.

It was in my DNA to know when an addict was lying, even when they were coordinating with friends to gaslight you. Flushing those pills down the toilet, I realized that I wasn't *saving* anyone—I was sinking. And as hard as we may try, addiction will never, ever be cured by love.

At the end of May, I told Jimmy I didn't want to marry him. He begged me to reconsider, asking if I'd go through with the wedding and then annul it, so that he wouldn't be made a fool of to his family and friends. I said he needed to get treatment. He swore, again, that he wasn't using. But I knew I had to leave—*really* leave—this time. I imagined having a kid with Jimmy, aware they'd grow up with the same terror and instability I lived with as a child, trauma I am, all these years later, still healing from. That kid wouldn't feel safe in their own home, as I hadn't. How heartless would I have to be to deprive a child of safety? In hindsight, it's distressing that I had to invent a child to cast my pain onto—that my own, tangible pain wasn't enough to get me to *go*.

I left with both our dogs in tow, packing into a tiny one-bedroom in Fort Greene that I drained my savings account to pay for, even with help from my parents for the broker fee. When I came back to the apartment I'd shared with Jimmy to collect my last few things, the dead bolt was locked and he wouldn't answer calls or texts. Later that week, he moved eighteen hundred miles away.

He called late one night around my twenty-eighth birthday in August, two months before our canceled wedding.

"I was taking pills," he said. "Then heroin. I went through withdrawal on the drive. I'm clean now."

Over the following months, he continued to contact me.

"It's the day we were supposed to get married," he texted on October 9. "You owe it to me to talk to me."

Jimmy wasn't a bad man. He just wasn't a good one, either.

For many years, I was fearful to tell anyone what was happening in my home with Jimmy. I despised their judgment and worried they'd call me a fool for staying—or worse, tell me that I'd made my bed. I couldn't bear hearing that I was "repeating the cycle" of my parents' marriage. Instead, the few close friends and family I disclosed to were kind, offering to do whatever it took to make me safe. As I was preparing to leave Jimmy, my managing editor at the *Beast* told me to take off the time I needed and that the rest of the team would pick up the slack just like they had when I was in the hospital. Their support made me brave in a way I wasn't able to be on my own.

When I canceled the wedding, I was consumed by shame. I'd been keeping so many secrets about my relationship, and I felt like I needed to explain *all* of them to *everyone* in order to defend my choice. (When you call off a wedding, everyone wants to know why. The first question isn't "How are you?" but rather "Why?") It was exhausting. Months later, I recognized that leaving Jimmy was perhaps the first decision I'd ever made that was for my well-being and my well-being *only*. And for a long time, that felt selfish. Until, eventually, I understood it was the kindest thing I've ever done for myself.

The physical process of moving on from Jimmy was easy: pack boxes, load truck, unload truck, unpack boxes, arrange, rearrange, learn the new noises and smells of the place, explore the neighborhood, find a good coffee shop, frequent the nearby dog park. But when I wasn't in motion, I hated myself. I worried that Jimmy would overdose and die. I wondered if the dogs missed him, and if I'd done the right thing taking them away from him. I remembered a couple of times that I had painkillers in the house after my hospitalizations, and I wished I'd locked them up or hid them; I never noticed any missing, but I also wasn't counting. I wondered if my carelessness had caused his relapse. Lying quietly in bed at night, I didn't know or like myself very much. But I felt safe, finally, and that safety allowed me to slowly start forgiving myself.

I forgave myself for repeating harmful patterns learned in childhood.

I forgave myself for thinking it was my job to fix another human.

I forgave myself for doing what I had to do to survive.

I forgave myself for isolating from friends and family.

I forgave myself for losing sight of who I am.

I forgave myself for being dishonest—outright or by omission—to hide abuse.

I forgave myself for believing bad men. (Okay, I'm still working on this one.)

Doc used to warn me about stress as an IBD trigger. He said that I could do everything else right—take my medication on time, see him regularly, eat the right stuff—but if I didn't control stress, I'd keep flaring. "The mind and the gut are intimately connected," he'd remind me. I shrugged, then kept working around the clock, checking the news on Twitter in the middle of the night, replying to emails on vacation, logging on to Slack, and editing features through the weekends. Most stressful of all, though, I remained with a man I was afraid of. I was constantly on high alert, trying to predict an unpredictable partner's moods and get in front of his aggression. Like I had as a child, I protected myself by becoming small.

Once I left Jimmy and truly felt safe, my health improved. I had a nasty bout of the chicken pox in the summer of 2016 and a short hospitalization for a Crohn's flare in early 2017, but it was remedied by an increased dosage of my biologic medication, which then got me into remission. Though I've had mild flares since then, I haven't been hospitalized for IBD since 2017. That seems monumental. (I feel like I'm going to jinx it just by writing about it!) I credit the right medication and dosage for getting me into my current long-term remission after five years of constant hospitalizations, in both long and short stretches. But my personal circumstances changed, too—secure living situation, stable relationship, less demanding work—in a way that positively contributes to my sustained physical and mental health.

"If you would have said to me back in 1982 that stress could modulate how the immune system worked, I would have said 'Forget about it,'" immunologist Dr. Ronald Glaser told the *New York Times* in 2002. Nearly twenty years after that quote, researchers are still scratching the surface in terms of understanding how the brain and the rest of the body communicate with each other, but there's no scientific doubt that they do. Stress doesn't have to feel huge, like that of an abusive relationship, to impact your body. Daily work stress (which you'll read more about in Chapter Fourteen), parenting, isolation, microaggressions, the news, managing finances—all of these life stressors worm their way into your brain and, in turn, your body, and when you're already chronically ill, they can make you feel significantly worse. Stress is inevitable, which is why managing it—through therapy, self-care, and strong social support—is so important.

CHAPTER 12

Friends

Chronic illness not only complicated my attitude toward family but also toward my friends. Rather than share how I felt in the wake of my diagnosis, I instinctively chose to isolate. In my early years with chronic illness, my friends needed me to explain the mechanics of IBD and how different it made my life, but explaining these things felt overwhelming and, ultimately, exhausting. I resented my friends for not educating themselves. I wanted them to read my mind and became angry when they couldn't. Plus, I was deeply ashamed to be young and sick, so I worried that my friends secretly pitied me. I questioned every text, every invitation: Are they doing this because they like me or because they feel bad for me? Add in uncontrolled anxiety and my desperate scrambling for control, and I was in a bad way.

"People sometimes don't disclose illness even to a close friend," Dr. Karen Winkler said. "They may want to be seen as strong and independent and fun, not the one who's complaining or having [chronic illness] symptoms. But all that hiding and non-disclosure can reinforce a shameful identity."

When I became ill, I bailed on dinners and brunches and birthday parties with little to no explanation. I was absent, I was aloof; then, I'd guilt-spiral for days. I know that had I communicated with my friends about my physical and mental illnesses, I would have been met with understanding and offers to help. But I failed to be open with them back then, and my distance must have been confusing and painful from the outside.

Now, on days when light is hard to come by, I turn to my community of chronically ill folks. A few years ago, I joined an online support group for women and femmes with IBD and ostomies. For a long time, I was too nervous to participate, so I spent weeks reading other members' posts and watching how the group responded. I quickly understood that this community cared for its members in the most loving way. There seemed to be an unwritten rule that this was a place without judgment, where members could be sick and feel, openly, all the complex emotions that come with chronic illness. It was a place to be *free*. I've since joined two other support groups, including an online community for people (and caretakers of people) who need the same biologic medication I do. As an infliximab veteran now, I spend most of my time there talking to new patients and caretakers, mostly moms of young IBDers, about their fears—the same ones I had before my first infusion. And even when I'm not interacting in my online support groups, just knowing they're there, full of people like me, dulls the lonely ache of forever sickness. Connecting with other chronically ill people teaches you how to carry each other's weight—when to lift when you have the strength, and when to share the burden when you have no energy left. I've found the chronic illness and disability community to be one of endless empathy and generosity.

But my openness to connecting did not come easy. For the

most part, life taught me to be wary of people, always anticipating them to leave or let me down. I learned to isolate and keep secrets. I couldn't ask for help, because who was going to help me? But chronic illness peeled back those defenses. It showed me that people do more than just hurt each other—they nurture, they listen, they enrich one another's lives. (It also made me brave enough to end the relationships that weren't beneficial to my well-being.) The ones who unconditionally love and support you can't remedy chronic illness, but they sure can make it easier to carry. As the psychiatrist and Holocaust survivor Viktor Frankl wrote, "Survival is a community event."

And though chronic illness initially made my friendships difficult to navigate, over time it gave me clarity about my toxic friendships. "Not every friendship is meant to support you in the same way. When you're chronically ill, you need to evaluate those friendships [and] understand how each friend can support you," Cohesive Therapy's Karen Conlon said during one of our several conversations. "Can I talk to this friend about heavy, deep issues? Do I trust them with personal information? What boundaries do I need to set with this friend? Don't spend your energy seeking out the friend who doesn't match the situation." It turned out that some of my friendships were not beneficial to my well-being and needed to end. I didn't always do this gracefully; I recognize now that endings deserve care and delicacy, even when you're hurt. But back then, I ended relationships the only way I knew how: I ghosted. "If you're feeling like a friend's response [to your illness] isn't validating, then there's a possibility that friend is having a hard time dealing with your situation," Conlon said. "A [difficult] conversation may be in order if you value that friendship."

Part of the reason friendships are so tricky to navigate is

because, as important as those relationships are, there's not a lot of guidance on how to get through the challenging parts; counseling is available for couples and families, but "friend therapy" isn't widely advertised. It's up to the people within the friendship to face the challenges together, dedicated enough to the relationship to try and fail. So how can healthy friends show up for their chronically ill pals? Most important, learn about your chronically ill friend's illness(es). "Education is key here. It's hard for a healthy person to understand what someone who's ill might be experiencing so education and communication are key," grief and loss counselor Diane Brennan said. "It might mean that the ill person needs to provide resources like websites, books, and YouTube videos to help someone understand that they can't just 'get over it.' This requires the ill person to communicate what they're experiencing and the [healthy] person to listen while suspending judgment."

When friends get educated about their chronically ill friend's disease(s), it becomes easier to know what the friend might need, which lightens the chronically ill friend's burden. "Be the friend who acknowledges that your friend's illness may need attention but is not a bother to you. Decenter yourself and be the friend who's mindful of the specifics, so that it doesn't always fall on the chronically ill friend to do the accommodating. When should we eat? Where should we eat? Are you okay to walk? I'm not sure that place has the best bathroom accessibility. Has your pain been low today? How about I bring food over and we stay in?" Dr. Winkler recommended. "You can be a good friend by taking the initiative to learn and read about the illness, and by letting your chronically ill friend know that you want to listen to what they're going through, if they're willing to share. And as a person with chronic illness, you can encourage your friends by telling them what would help *you* for them to know, and expressing appreciation that they're trying to understand." I would add: Be the friend who listens to the chronically ill people in your life, not the friend who tries to minimize or fix the situation. Don't offer unsolicited advice. *Just listen.*

And chronically ill people can still show up for their friends, even when they can't be around physically. Check in via text and email. Set up Facetime dates. Ask if they're in the right headspace to talk about heavy stuff before dumping it on them (this goes both ways in a friendship). And make an effort to discuss something other than your illness; ask about their work, their families, their own physical and mental health. Laugh with each other! It doesn't have to feel weird or awkward just because one of you is chronically ill. You still have the same needs as any other friends: to feel connected, loved, supported; to laugh, to vent, to listen.

When I started to write about my illness, something shifted in how I thought about friendships. Sharing—in effect, releasing the control I was trying to gather by isolating and secret-keeping—made me brave. Shaky at first but brave nonetheless. Posting online gave me a protective barrier, like dipping my toe in a swimming pool to test the temperature. Right around the time I started writing about my illness, I also became friends with people in online IBD support groups. And as I continued to share through writing and build friendships virtually, talking IRL about my physical and mental illnesses became less of a big deal. Shame began to dissolve. So, yes, the internet is a hellhole filled with misogynists and right-wing extremists, but it's also a vital channel for chronically ill people to connect with one another and the greater world—making our lives brighter and fuller, even on the days when our worlds extend no further than a hospital room. The definition of what makes a "real" friend dissolves when your world shrinks due to chronic illness—online friends *are* our real friends. (You know how you felt about the internet as a vital channel during COVID-19 isolation? That's how chronically ill and disabled people feel about it all the time!)

By the time I got terribly sick in 2015, I wasn't afraid to post health updates on social media. On the lowest days, I asked for good vibes—every "like" was someone sending me their best. It seems silly, but it helped to know that people cared about me even enough to click. These gestures felt like some kind of collective support behind my recovery, and that made me stronger when I wanted to just give up and die. As the weeks wore on, it became increasingly hard for me to have any perspective outside of Methodist's bubble, and those online interactions, no matter how small, kept me connected to the outside world. People I barely knew beyond the realm of the internet sent me emails and DMs, but also letters, cards, flowers, and trinkets to my hospital room.

My colleagues at the *Daily Beast*, where I was an editor at the time, organized the entire newsroom to hand-draw cards for me; some people made cartoons, comic strips, crayon drawings, even watercolors. My managing and executive editors emailed me weekly to check in—not in a "when are you getting back to work" way but a "we care about you" way; my staff writers sent office gossip and funny observations to lift my spirits. Our international editor lit candles for me in churches around the world, a particularly comforting gesture even though I'm not religious. I've never known such kindness as that which was shown to me that spring. The way people treat you when you're chronically ill will break your heart repeatedly—sometimes in the excruciating way, and sometimes in the remarkable way.

Social support is paramount for chronically ill people not only because it increases the opportunity for growth and can decrease symptoms of depression and anxiety but because it offsets the risk of loneliness and isolation, which chronically ill people are at high risk for. Chronic loneliness—meaning an ongoing lack of social connections—comes with serious physical and mental health effects, and in recent years there's been a push to consider loneliness a public health issue. Here's some of what we know, via the National Institute on Aging:[1]

- Loneliness increases the risk of depression.
- Loneliness also increases the risk of cognitive decline in older adults.
- Loneliness ups your risk of high blood pressure, heart disease, decreased immune function, and poor sleep.
- Loneliness is associated with low self-esteem, poor coping skills, and the inability to perform daily tasks.
- In old age, loneliness increases the risk of self-harm and suicide.

It's also true that you can be alone and not feel lonely, or that you can be surrounded by loved ones and *still* feel the ache of loneliness. Loneliness is a complex psychological and physical

---

1. "Featured Research: Social Isolation, Loneliness in Older People Pose Health Risks," US Department of Health & Human Services: National Institute on Aging, last updated April 23, 2019; accessed April 10, 2020, https://www.nia.nih.gov/news/social-isolation-loneliness-older-people-pose-health-risks.

issue that researchers don't understand entirely but suspect has genetic and environmental influences (and, it doesn't seem that being an introvert or an extrovert shields you from feeling lonely). What we do know is that feeling a sense of connection to your community when you're chronically ill impacts how you think about your own illness, including how positive you are about the future, how understood you feel, and how supported you believe you are through extended periods of illness.

CHAPTER 13

A Pox

I was eating dinner with my now-husband Greg on a humid July night when I felt the first blister. The 2016 election was forthcoming and everyone in the city could talk about little else. Greg and I hadn't known each other long and were in the early days of dating but had figured out almost instantly that we were in love. I tend to touch my face a lot when I speak—a nervous thing—so my fingers grazed my left cheek, tracing the bone to where it meets the jaw, just below the ear. I discovered a small, tender bump. It popped when I pressed it, leaving clear fluid on my fingertips. I felt another one just above my right eyebrow. *Pop.* The next day, hundreds of the little red blisters speckled my face, shoulder blades, chest, and groin. I snapped pictures of the spots and sent them to Greg and Mom: "Holy shit."

They itched incessantly, but even worse, every red dot sent a sharp, shooting pain into the muscle and bone beneath it. Each bump felt deeply tethered to the layers of flesh below, like a plant to its roots. This was nerve pain, the emergency room doctor explained, a signature symptom of varicella zoster, the virus that causes chicken pox.

Fucking *chicken pox.*

A week earlier, I'd gone to a walk-in clinic for a urinary tract infection I couldn't kick, and a child, eight or nine years old, in the waiting room had the rash. I jokingly sent a text to Greg: "There's a kid here with chicken pox. Knowing my luck, I'll get it!" Well.

Usually, varicella is spread through close contact (i.e., the blisters themselves), but it can also spread via air—a cough or sneeze from someone who's infected—or a contaminated surface. It's easy for people with compromised immune systems to catch, and dangerous. See, healthy immune systems not only try to protect you from getting sick in the first place, they also help fight off bugs when you do catch something. But when your immune system is actively suppressed, like mine, it can't protect you well from getting sick in the first place; then, when it's supposed to fight an invader, it sputters but doesn't start. Chicken pox puts even healthy adults at risk for serious complications like pneumonia and meningitis, though for most, it remedies in a week to ten days.

I fought the goddamn chicken pox for almost three months. (Vaccinate your kids, people.)

The first couple of weeks were miserable. My fever stayed high and I was constantly itchy and sore. The antiviral medication valacyclovir (the same stuff used to treat herpes—chicken pox, shingles, cold sores, and genital herpes are all related) made me queasy. As one patch of spots would crust, a new patch would pop up. Greg changed my cold washcloths and gently dabbed my spots with calamine lotion. He held me up to take sips of Gatorade. He even put the bedsheets in the freezer to help cool me down. I slept day and night, waking only to check my temperature and apply calamine lotion. I later asked Greg why he took such around-the-clock care of me when we barely knew each other. "Because I loved you," he said.

I blamed myself for getting the chicken pox, of course. It all goes back to when I went to youth group at age thirteen. Mom and Dad had recently split up and I was seeking something—stability, probably, and rebellion against my nonreligious-occasionally-Buddhist dad. My town was small, white, and conservative, which meant there was a church on every block. I chose the biggest, loudest one: the Baptist church. The Baptists were scriptural literalists who taught me a lot over the following years, such as: salvation is the sole way to heaven, virginity is a girl's most prized possession, NSYNC is the devil's music, girls should only hug boys sideways so the boys can avoid contact with those wicked breasts, Catholics are probably going to hell and Buddhists are *definitely* going to hell, gayness can be cured, man is the head of the church and the household, the Bible is the one book anyone needs to read (and really, only men need to read it), we have to pray for George W. Bush, and unborn babies are the Lord's army and must be protected at all costs. In the church, girls and women were not complex beings. We were virgins or whores; the virgins grew up to be mild-mannered wives and mothers while the whores existed to lead men astray.

I was invested for about two years—long enough to be baptized and go on a mission trip to the Bahamas where my only qualification was being white—before I snapped out of it. This brand of religion was and is toxic, hypocritical, and rooted in white supremacy, sexism, and homophobia. In return for my time with the church, I got a lot of free pizza and a good look at everything I never want to be as a human. But there are two things that have stuck with me from those years: one, an encyclopedia of hymns that pop into my head at completely inappropriate moments, like when my dog finally poops after sniffing six hundred spots in twenty-degree weather. *"Our God is an awesome God / He reigns from Heaven above / With wisdom, power, and love / Our God is an awesome God!"* And, two, this idea that we're punished for our sins. Though I had long abandoned allegiance to any higher power, I thought the chicken pox might be the universe's karmic punishment for leaving Jimmy and soon after falling in love with Greg, similar to how it'd crossed my mind that Crohn's could be my penalty for letting Dad die on the toilet. In a backward way, I was almost glad that with the chicken pox, my "punishment" was visible, a kind of biblical plague of boils. I realize this is an irrational line of thinking, but sometimes brains deal with things in illogical ways.

Reality is less apocalyptic. I don't have much control over my body. For unknown reasons, my immune system overreacts and attacks my digestive system. It has to be suppressed via medication to stop doing that. Suppressing my immune system means I catch viruses and bacterial infections easily, and then it's hard to get rid of them once I have them. I went to a walk-in clinic and wound up with chicken pox because I happened to be there at the same time as an unvaccinated kid. I was born to one abusive man and almost married another. *Que sera sera.*

Around week three with the chicken pox, Greg found a spot on his stomach and another on his face. His mom, when he called her, couldn't remember if he'd had the rash as a child. And since he was in his twenties by the time the chicken pox vaccine came around, he never got the shot. So, just a few weeks after meeting, we were both down with adult chicken pox. While Greg didn't get many spots, he was slammed with fever and aches for a week straight. But then, he felt better.

I, meanwhile, had to be hospitalized. Each time I finished a course of antiviral meds, the rash came back in new patches. My immune system wasn't picking up the slack, so the infectious disease doctor at Methodist (the same one I'd butted heads with in 2015—we came to understand each other a bit better this time) recommended I be hospitalized and put on stronger IV antivirals. I was isolated, of course, and any staff who hadn't already had chicken pox had to be gloved, masked, and gowned to enter the room. I knew some of the nurses and other staff from my IBD-related stays, and they couldn't believe my bad luck. "You're too young to be so sick all the time," they'd say. Next to my bed was a giant air filter that sucked up the potentially pox-contaminated air and filtered it elsewhere; its loud hum helped me sleep. I spent a week there, eating pudding and watching the Rio Olympics, before the doctor cleared me to continue antiviral pills at home. Still, it took another several weeks of medication and a slow taper before I stopped sprouting new spots.

I have chicken pox scars across my chest and shoulder blades that have faded into white, scattered stars. A deep, perfectly round one above my right eyebrow pisses me off every time I catch it in the mirror because it's a reminder that my world is smaller than it used to be, and that while I've come to terms with my chronic illness, I will always be at risk.

See, IBD shrank my world twice: once, upon my initial diagnosis, and again when I started infliximab. The disease itself forces me to be near a bathroom when I'm flaring, and even

when I'm not flaring if it decides to be unexpectedly temper-
amental. I'm almost always fatigued, on good days and bad. I
have to chart my course before I leave the house. I pack extra
underwear everywhere I go. I've skipped more professional and
social events than I care to count because it's easier not to go
than to plan for all the *what-ifs*. And I worry about where I'll
live in the future if I leave New York—will it be near a good hospital? Will the state protect my right to health care? Will I find
a doctor who understands me? I'd be sad to leave New York for
one hundred reasons, but most of all, to leave Doc.

Infliximab, the biologic drug that I started taking in 2015
under Doc and Dr. G.'s supervision, got me into remission in
just a few rounds, but the limitations of what I could do safely
grew even smaller. Infliximab works on the idea that people
with Crohn's disease have too much tumor necrosis factor alpha
(TNF-alpha), a protein that regulates immune cells.[1] An abun-
dance of TNF causes the immune system to overreact, leading
to inflammation, so infliximab blocks it. For some patients, it
works for a long time, but others build antibodies and have to
switch to another biologic or different treatment. I get tested for
antibodies at least once a year and, thankfully, haven't developed
any yet.

Infliximab came with the chance of side effects, some not so
serious and some very serious. The latter included drug-induced
lupus, activation of hepatitis B and tuberculosis in people who
already have those diseases, increased risk of melanoma, ana-
phylaxis, stroke, and lymphoma, a cancer of the lymphatic
system—an important part of the immune system that includes
lymph nodes, bone marrow, spleen, and thymus gland—that

---

1. "What Is Remicade?," Janssen CarePath, last updated 2019; accessed February
3, 2020, https://www.remicade.com/crohns-disease/learn-about-remicade.html.

can spread to other organs. Dr. G. told me that about six in ten thousand people who take anti-TNF agents get lymphoma.[2] In all likelihood, I wouldn't get cancer, though it was still a frightening prospect. But I was so desperate to feel better that my thought process was, *If I get cancer, I'll deal with it then.*

Chronically ill people make decisions like this all the time. We so badly want sustained health that we choose treatments with serious, even life-threatening, side effects. The alternative is to *not feel better*, so we cross our fingers and hope for the best. When you're healthy, you can take your time with choices, weighing them carefully. But when you're sick, you have tunnel vision. You're in survival mode. The options are either keep feeling bad, or try a thing that might *or* might not work, and might *or* might not make you feel better (*or* might make you feel worse). So, we try the thing.

At first, infliximab's side effects were rough—plus, I was still very much recovering from several months of IBD flaring and *C. diff*. With time, the side effects lessened or went away with the exception of two: ocular migraines every fifteen days, without fail, and psoriasis in odd places like my left earlobe, the top of my butt crack, and my belly button. (Psoriasis can progress in places of injury: an ear piercing, a long-abandoned belly button piercing, and, well, we all know my behind has had a rough few years.)

But the worst part about infliximab is that, because it suppresses my immune system, it makes me more prone to infections. It's the reason why my bout with the chicken pox lasted three months—and why when I get colds, flus, and other bugs, they last longer than they would if I had a fully functioning

2. https://www.sciencedirect.com/science/article/abs/pii/S1542356509000524.

immune system. The first year of my infusions, I got a urinary tract infection every month even though I was doing everything right: peeing after sex, wiping front to back, staying hydrated, not holding it when I needed to go. It was maddening. During flu season, I barely leave the apartment. My brain zooms in on surfaces, like the handle of a grocery cart, as I imagine how many germs are there waiting to make me sick. (You can imagine my mental state during a pandemic.) And IBD patients can't take NSAIDs, so no ibuprofen to help the symptoms of one of those colds or flus. I can't get live vaccines or boosters, and because of my weakened immune system combined with my *C. diff* risk, I can't take antibiotics unless the reason for them outweighs the chance of recurrence.

Everything has become a cost/benefit analysis: *Is it worth getting [a cold, the flu, fill in the blank] if I go?* I'm likely to get sick from going to parties, concerts, airports, subways, and offices, and then it takes me much longer than a healthy, non-immune-suppressed person to recover. One party can mean weeks of illness. When I was still working in a newsroom, I took car services to avoid the subway—"a germ tunnel," Doc called it—but this got untenably expensive, so I bought a cheap used car instead. I spent more in parking tickets than the car was worth. Then, I sold the car to pay for my wisdom teeth extraction. I skipped even more social and work events. I passed up travel because I didn't want to wear a mask and gloves on the plane and have everyone stare (though in a post-COVID society, now we stare at the folks *not* wearing masks), and I didn't want to be away from my doctors in case I needed them. I hated all the life changes chronic illness had forced me to make, and somewhere in my brain, I still blamed myself for getting sick in the first place.

Blame is a natural part of grieving a loss, and as I wrote in Chapter Five, it's a way to cling to hope. If we're able to find something that caused an illness, that reinforces a sense of order in the world. It means there's a definite cause, and if there's a cause, there must be a cure. Blame leaves room for that possibility. But when illness happens for no reason other than "genetics and environment," and there is no cure, the desired sense of order is thrown to the wind. I once saw this on a bereavement card: "Shit doesn't have to make sense." And it's stuck with me. I used to think there was some kind of cap on pain—that once a person had hit a certain level of hurt, they wouldn't have any more. "God doesn't give you more than you can handle," as the saying goes. But that isn't the way it works at all. Some people have more suffering, and some have less, and there's no rhyme or reason why. Bad stuff happens to good people with no other explanation than *it just happens*. Little babies die suddenly and horrible old billionaires live to see 105 and decent people get sick forever. Shit will never make sense.

For hundreds of years, health problems were ascribed to moral failings. Sick people weren't right with God, and illness, be it individual or widespread, was due to human sin. (Some Evangelical sects still preach this.) It's no coincidence that the poorest communities were the sickest. Wealthy citizens and politicians could ignore any investment in public health so long as illness was a problem of the soul, not the society. They'd retire to their country estates—in essence, quarantining themselves—during outbreaks of sickness in cities. When they avoided illness, it further reinforced wealth and health as connected to superior

moral standing. This didn't last forever, though. As city populations grew and rich and poor lived in closer proximity, wealthy
families got sick and died just as poor ones did. And when that
happened, people in power started to pay more attention (and in
turn, give more money) to public health systems.

Though science has progressed since then to show that illness spreads via bacteria, virus, or genetics and not because of
godlessness, there's still a lingering idea that sick people—and
poor people—have failed in some way, that they're somehow
unclean or unworthy, bringing this suffering upon themselves.
That line of thinking makes it easier to withhold health care
from the people who need it most. We saw this phenomenon
with COVID-19. A public "othering" happened: *Only* the
elderly were at risk of dying. *Only* immune-compromised people
were seriously fucked. *Only* poor people without the resources to
shelter in place would get it. (We now know that none of this is
true, anyway. Young, healthy people got very sick and died from
COVID-19.)

We forever-sick folks internalize the "othering" until it becomes
very loud. *Maybe I did do something to bring this upon myself.
Maybe I don't deserve to feel better—or live. Maybe I am worthless.* This inner dialogue was prevalent when I saw myself in the
mirror covered with hundreds of red spots, irredeemably disgusting. Even when the pox faded, there was still something
invisibly gross and wrong about me, I thought. Thoughts like
these get reinforced by the fact that chronic illness—particularly
one as unsexy as bowel disease—is not a popular topic of conversation. It makes people uncomfortable. And so chronically
ill people feel ashamed. We split ourselves in two trying to keep
people around us *comfortable*—and sometimes, the hiding feels
as exhausting as the illness itself.

Similar judgments crept in during the COVID pandemic as I considered just how many people—even those I know personally—would sacrifice my well-being for a haircut or to eat in a restaurant. What a strange historical moment to live through, when I can turn on the TV or open Instagram and hear politicians or see acquaintances argue why my life and lives like mine are less important than the good of the Dow. "We can't let the cure be worse than the problem itself" (the president); "As a senior citizen, are you willing to take a chance on your survival in exchange for keeping America and all that America loves for your children and grandchildren? . . . I'm all in" (Texas lieutenant governor Dan Patrick); and "In the choice between the loss of our way of life as Americans and the loss of life, of American lives, we have to always choose the latter" (Indiana representative Trey Hollingsworth). *All lives matter, right guys?!* I don't believe them about anything, of course, but it's still distressing. (Ableism, I should note, is pervasive across the political spectrum. When Donald Trump did something dumb or evil or both, which was all the time, social media lit up with speculation that he was riddled with dementia or Parkinson's or whatever armchair diagnosis was popular that day. People like to ascribe physical and mental ailments to cruel men rather than accepting that they are just that: cruel men.)

On a lighter note, I want to say one last thing about blaming. You know who will have the wisdom to never, ever blame you for being sick? Your dog.

When chronically ill people write to ask for my advice, I tell them two things: First, find a good therapist or support group (or, ideally, both!). And second, if you're able, get a dog. Or get two dogs! But don't get four like I have. Four is entirely too many dogs—though in my defense, it happened by accident. I had two and Greg had two and then we fell in love and . . . wait a second. This is the dog version of *The Brady Bunch*.

These four silly, stinky, adoring dogs contribute to my well-being every day. (If you're wondering how we've managed so many dogs in New York City, the answer is: with humor.) My day-to-day life revolves around their care and feeding and affection, making sure I honor their individual personalities and quirks, remembering that they're dogs, not humans. They snap me out of my self-loathing by doing something goofy, they make me get fresh air several times a day because I have to walk them even when I'd rather hide indoors, and they stick by my side on high pain days. Can dogs sense when we're sick? I'm not sure, but I like to think they've been hanging out with humans for so many thousands of years now that the answer is yes. Virginia Woolf, who was mentally and physically ill for most of her life, wrote, "Half the horrors of illness cease when one has a book or a dog or a cup of one's own at hand."

The scientific benefits of having a pet around are long established, too. Florence Nightingale, credited as the founder of modern nursing, touted dogs as beneficial for wounded soldiers' healing processes. Sigmund Freud, love him or hate him, was known to bring his beloved chow chows to patient sessions because he observed the dogs' calming effect on people. And when it comes to chronic illness, studies show that pets—be they dogs, cats, birds, horses, even reptiles—have a pain-reducing and mood-boosting effect. They also increase positive social behaviors and physical activity, lower blood pressure, and decrease stress. AIDS patients who have pets report less depression, and heart attack patients who have pets show longer survival rates.

These dogs will, in all likelihood, die before me. I don't mean to be macabre—that's just how canine life expectancy works. I'm aware all the time of their sped-up hourglass (sometimes I cry in the shower thinking about them dying before me, which Greg says I should try to stop doing), and so I'm always looking for things to please them, new experiences, interesting foods they haven't tried. If I can't always be good and kind to myself, I can always be good and kind to these dogs. They rely on me—and that makes it difficult to get wrapped up in my own neuroses for any length of time. They also care for me in that wordless canine way, shadowing my every move when I don't feel well, nuzzling my face when I cry. They aren't judgmental of the days I can't get out of bed—instead, they're happy to nap alongside me, curling up in the curve of my abdomen like little living heating pads. They have no idea that I have a book deal and wouldn't love me any more even if they did. They're always so excited when they wake up and realize nothing changed while they were asleep and they get to do another day—even if it's the same as every other day before that. I learn a lot from them.

Our dogs are called Gixer, Lady, Fievel, and Dolly. Dolly, the baby of the family, a shy black and tan Shiba Inu, is suspicious of all new people but hugely loving to me and to Greg, her human soul mate. She comes alive in nature and once heroically sniffed out my father-in-law's lost hearing aid in the red-dirt mountains of North Carolina. I've watched her personality come alive more every year—from a scared, trembling lump of fur to a fearless explorer—and it reminds me every day that, even if I do fall into a bad habit and blame myself for things over which I have no control, as the poet Rainer Maria Rilke wrote, "No feeling is final."

CHAPTER 14

Work

When I was diagnosed with IBD, one of my greatest and most immediate fears was how the illness would impact my career. Without realizing it, I'd wrapped up my self-worth with how rapidly I could climb the ladder. At twenty-three, I was an editor at Lifehacker, and I thought that said *something* about me, something more than how I made money. To me, it proved who I was as a person. "See how young and successful I am?! See this blue checkmark on my Twitter account?!" If everyone else thought I was doing well, then I felt like I *was* doing well. The illusion mattered more to me than the committed, hard work required for true well-being.

When I was the sickest I've ever been that spring of 2015, my self-designated marker of "health" was getting back to work as an editor at the *Daily Beast*. After a long leave of absence, my celebratory "I'm back!" Facebook post said, "I just turned off my out of office message!" Returning to work was supposed to mean everything was back to normal—but a year later in 2016, I left the job entirely. I couldn't work long hours anymore and deal with stress stirring up my symptoms. A lot of days, I had to take opiate painkillers just to handle the discomfort from hours sitting at my desk. And, frankly, I didn't feel as invested in the work as I once had.

So, I made the tough choice to give up employer-based health insurance and a steady income for the tightrope of freelancing. And it wasn't like things were perfect at the *Beast*, despite the camaraderie of my colleagues and the kindness shown to me during my hospitalizations. The demand for content caused people to make big mistakes, like an infamous 2016 story where a straight reporter baited gay Olympians via dating apps; higher-ups emailed and texted us at all hours, seven days a week; the reporters who most deserved raises never got them; when staff left for other jobs, they were often guilted and treated terribly; people had panic attacks in the bathroom and cried at their desks, and we all became so accustomed to it that we thought it was normal. In the weeks after I came back to work post–chicken pox, my budget was slashed to $1,200/month (10 percent of what I'd started with) and management would publish one or two of my vertical's story a week compared to two or more a day prior. I knew I was being forced out, but I didn't care. I was ready to leave. I freelanced for several months before totally freaking out about money and health insurance, and in August 2017, I hastily took a job as an editor at a women's magazine.

But there's something that happens in health and wellness media that no one really speaks about: Outlets will gladly publish stories about the trauma of living with chronic illness. Readers love war stories. But when it comes to employing chronically ill and disabled folks and accommodating our needs, media bosses are less enthusiastic. I disclosed my illness to my magazine boss shortly after I was hired; it was unavoidable since I had to miss full days in the office for treatment, though I still worked from the infusion center. Seeing as we were a publication focused on health and intersectional feminism, I expected my boss to be obliging—or thankful, even, to have someone on staff with my experience and perspective. Instead, she became cold, dismissive, and infantilizing. I was on the verge of a panic attack every morning and relied on benzodiazepines more than I'd have liked. I lost ten pounds and couldn't sleep. I agonized over every interaction with my manager, which made my work suffer and led to dumb mistakes. I lasted four months before quitting.

In the process, I discovered that something glorious happens after you've come close to death: You stop giving a fuck. Or, it would be more accurate to say: You stop giving a fuck about the shit that doesn't matter and start giving a fuck about what does. I didn't want to spend one more second worrying about office politics, pageviews, publishing quotas, or passive-aggressive bosses. No more watered-down coffee, $16 cafeteria salads, and antianxiety pills just to make it to my desk every morning. No more *open fucking office plan*. I would hunker down and figure out a way to make a decent living via freelancing, where I could make my own schedule and be my own manager and do the work that I wanted to. I could be fully in my body on good days and bad, without sneaking around a boss who sees me less as a person and more as a pageview producer. I could turn my phone off at bedtime and not check my email first thing in the morning, panicked about deadlines and assignments and news cycles. I would be free of the daily anxiety shits. *HUZZAH!*

This was, shall we say, optimistic. Freelancing doesn't mean you're suddenly able to do the work you want 24/7—it means you do the work you *have* to do to pay the bills, and every so often, get to do a passion project. Anyone who tells you that money doesn't buy happiness has never been hungry or had the lights shut off or had to skip medical treatment—and they definitely haven't known the stomach-gnawing fear that comes with late paychecks when you make decisions like *I guess I'll skip buying groceries to pay the [fill in the blank] bill.* Work-related anxiety doesn't go away, it just shifts from, say, your boss, to managing your schedule, pitching stories, lining up other work, invoicing clients, and wrangling paychecks. It's always going to be stressful paying for health insurance. And I'm always going to be hooked on the news cycle because I have an insatiable need to know what's going on in the world.

But I've created boundaries now that didn't exist before. I don't sleep with my phone under my head in case a story breaks, and I removed the Twitter app from my smartphone (and then re-downloaded it during the shelter in place order, and then deleted it again). Because I can make my own schedule, my physical and mental health have both improved. I work from home, and on days when I need extra rest, I work from bed or take the day off, making up the work later when I feel better. I even work from the bathtub when I'm in a lot of pain. I never worry about spending too much time in the bathroom, and I can move my schedule around for doctors' appointments and infusions. Plus, I've worked it out to where I usually have a paycheck every fifteen days, which reduces the financial stress some. Occasionally, I miss the camaraderie of a newsroom, and I'm mindful that the isolation of working from home can negatively affect my mental health. And I have no steady salary to fall back on. Though I haven't had a serious flare-up since I began freelancing in 2018, I'd lose a massive amount of income if I did. (After all, if I'm not working, I'm not making money.) Still, it's a great privilege to be able to work the way I do.

Coming close to death forced me to reevaluate not only what I could physically and mentally handle, but what I wanted the rest of my life to look like. In a turn of events I never could have predicted, I started caring *less* about the work and *more* about my body. After years of Doc reminding me how stress would negatively impact my disease, I understood in the lead-up to the 2016 election that he was right—I could no longer work long, tense hours in an always-on newsroom. So when I caught the chicken pox a few months before election day, I started planning my *Beast* exit. In the slow hospital hours, I made pros and cons lists. *Pro: Less stress; Con: Less money. Pro: Make my own schedule; Con: Accountable only to myself. Pro: Time off for sick days and doctors' appointments; Con: No health insurance. Pro: Predictable salary; Con: Financial free fall.*

You can see from that list that my biggest fears were financial. Like a lot of chronically ill people, my ability to afford health insurance—and thus, to stay well—was tied to my employment, and it was unsettling to think about life without that safety net. As a freelancer I could sign up for health insurance through the marketplace—but what if I was too sick to work and couldn't afford that payment? Chronically ill folks in America are wholly aware of this harsh truth: Lack of money makes us sick(er) and being sick(er) leads to lack of money. That snake eating its own tail was branded on my brain as I tried to decide how—and if I even could—leave my job and strike out on my own. (I'm lucky that my chosen field even allows for such a consideration.)

I dealt with the worst years of my illness in demanding jobs, and it taught me a lot: how to deal with understanding and not-so-understanding bosses and colleagues, how to take a leave of absence, and how to decipher confusing health insurance options. I learned on the fly because I had to. But, if I could go back and tell my younger self anything, here's what I'd pass along:

It's your choice whether you disclose your illness or not— but you might want to.

It's nerve-racking to tell your boss that you're chronically ill and that your illness might require adjustments to the way you work. A thousand questions run through your head: Will this put my job at risk? Will my boss think I'm unreliable or regret hiring me? Will my colleagues resent me for working from home or taking time off? Will this affect my ability to get a job recommendation in the future? On the other hand, disclosing your illness can feel freeing and will, hopefully, open up communication between you and your employer. And ideally, your boss will work to accommodate your needs. Disclosing your illness also prevents having to explain later on if your symptoms affect your job performance or attendance. But some chronically ill people choose not to tell their employer, and I understand that choice if they feel that it puts their job at risk. (Though it's illegal to fire an employee for an illness or disability, it still happens all the time, as do other discriminatory practices. Some disabled and chronically ill folks end up quitting work because the discrimination—be it overt or covert—becomes unbearable. Legal recourse, then, is expensive, financially and emotionally.)

I'm lucky that my illness can be hidden if I want it to be—that's a privilege folks with visible illnesses and disabilities or those who use mobility devices don't have. Still, it's been difficult to cloak my illness even when it's in remission since I've had to take days off for treatment, and because my personal and professional lives often overlap via writing. I've pursued jobs, then needed to delay the hiring process or turn down offers because of my health status. My medications caused noticeable side effects that I've felt warranted an explanation in the past. Plus, I don't feel like I *should* have to keep my illness a secret. My work requires a somewhat "public self," and I speak about my illness on social media. It's a big part of who I am and why I do the work I do, and my perspective should be a benefit to my employer, not a liability. Keeping my illness a secret makes it seem dishonorable, and I'm not ashamed to be chronically ill. Some bosses have been understanding and supportive when I've explained what Crohn's disease is, how it works, and the ways I manage it. Others have not. It's difficult to predict how even the most progressive-seeming managers will react to this disclosure.

You're the only one who can decide whether to reveal your illness or not—and legally, you don't have to. Employers can't ask about chronic illnesses or disabilities during an interview, and you aren't required to share before or after you're hired. But if you're going to disclose it, there are a few guidelines you should follow. First, understand the protections you have by law. The Americans with Disabilities Act (ADA) requires companies with more than fifteen employees provide "reasonable" accommodations to employees who disclose a disability;[1] it also protects job seekers who haven't been hired yet. Disability is defined in the law as "a physical or mental impairment that substantially limits one or more major life activities." A 2008 amendment broadened the definition to qualify illnesses that are episodic—e.g., flare-ups and remissions—or controlled with medication.[2] It also covers chronic illnesses that progress from manageable to debilitating.

If you request reasonable accommodations—say, working from home as needed, modifying your schedule, rearranging an office for wheelchair use, or providing unlimited bathroom access—and your employer denies them, they can face legal action, so it's in their best interest to provide what you need. Confidentially negotiating these accommodations can be done through human

---

1. "Fact Sheet: Disability Discrimination," US Equal Employment Opportunity Commission; accessed February 3, 2020, https://www.eeoc.gov/eeoc/publications/fs-ada.cfm.

2. Americans with Disabilities Act Amendments Act of 2008, Pub. L. 110-325 (January 1, 2009).

resources or a trained ADA mediator[3]—or with the help of a labor lawyer. Remember, at the end of the day, human resources exists to protect the company. If you feel like HR isn't representing your best interests, it might be time to bring in outside counsel. If you need a place to start, the National Disability Rights Network is a large nonprofit organization that, among other things, helps people with disabilities find legal services. You can also consult with your union or guild if you have one, or contact the Equal Employment Opportunity Commission (EEOC), a government agency that protects employees against discrimination and harassment, or file an ADA complaint with the Department of Justice. (You may have heard of the Occupational Safety and Health Administration, which is another government agency in place to protect workers. However, OSHA handles *on-the-job* illnesses and injuries, and we're talking about non-job-related chronic illnesses and disabilities here.)

Next, prepare for what you need to say and anticipate the questions you might be asked. You want your boss to understand that while your disease affects your life, you're still capable of doing your job. Deliver the necessary facts about your illness without bombarding your boss with information—keep it direct and simple. Be clear about how you manage the illness and that although you do your best to keep it under control, it can flare up. Tell your boss what you'll do if and when that happens. (If your disease is in remission, it can be helpful to mention that during this conversation. You can say something like, "My disease is in remission currently, and as long as my medication keeps working and I manage my lifestyle, it should remain that way for the foreseeable

---

3. "The ADA Mediation Program: Questions and Answers," US Department of Justice Civil Rights Division Disability Rights Section, last updated September 2016; accessed September 23, 2020, https://www.ada.gov/mediation_docs/mediation-q-a.htm.

future. But diseases like mine can be unpredictable, so here's the plan I have in place should I have a flare-up.") If you need days off for doctor's appointments or treatment, explain that to your boss, and if you can, get those days on the schedule as far in advance as possible. It might also be helpful to have a letter from your doctor that explains your illness.

I believe it's also important to explain how your illness makes you better at your work—for example, I have compassion for the chronically ill folks I write about because I understand them in a way that a non-chronically-ill journalist can't. I'm exceptionally adaptable. My perspective as a chronically ill woman is of value to a newsroom, and I'm connected to a giant readership that's been overlooked by most publishers. Remind your boss that your illness might change *how* you work, but it doesn't change *how well* you do your work. And take it from me, good work can happen from the bathtub. The COVID-19 pandemic has proven that flexible, remote work is doable; I hope the media industry learns a lesson from this and stops making jobs—underpaid ones at that—available *only* in the most expensive cities in the world. (I hope we demand other changes from this as well, building on the work started by chronically ill and disabled activists long before I was born: employment equity, stronger job security, mutual aid, the expansion of telehealth, internet as a public utility, harm reduction, decriminalization of drugs, accessible public spaces, health services over prisons, at-home instead of institutionalized care, and housing and health care for all. What's the greater point of this tragedy if we don't create a better world from it?)

During the interview process, you'll also want to come prepared with a list of your own questions that uncover how well a company treats its employees with illnesses and disabilities. This can get a little tricky if you're trying not to disclose your illness, but I suggest asking about paid sick leave, company policies about extended time off and remote work, and what the company did to protect and assist its employees during the COVID-19 pandemic (the answer to this question will reveal a lot).

What if my colleagues resent me for, say, working from home?

Fuck 'em.

(Okay, maybe that's not the most diplomatic answer. But truly: Fuck 'em.)

You don't owe an explanation about your illness to anyone in your workplace except your boss and HR should you decide to disclose, period. But if you feel like you need to explain why you're working from home one day a week or leaving often for doctor's appointments, here are a few points to keep in mind: First, decide who you're going to tell. You don't need to send a company-wide email, but you might want to let your immediate team know what's going on. Then, decide how much information you want to share. It can be as simple as, "Hi team, I'm dealing with an ongoing health issue and will be working from home every Friday. I'll be reachable there via Slack, phone, and email. If you want further details, I'm happy to discuss over coffee!" (Or not—you don't have to discuss anything further.) That message lets your coworkers feel informed without giving more information than you're comfortable sharing. Most people will wish you the best and leave it at that.

But what if you run into an office bully? You know, someone who demands to know why you get "special" accommodations when you don't even look sick? Say it with me: FUCK 'EM. Recognize that this kind of behavior comes from two things: personal unhappiness that has nothing to do with you, and a fundamental lack of understanding about what chronic illness is. You can't do anything about the first, but the second can be remedied with either an email or an in-person talk that explains what your illness is, how it affects your life, and why work accommodations help you. Simply saying, "I don't take a lot of bathroom breaks because I'm lazy. I take them because I have Crohn's disease, an incurable illness that causes my immune system to attack my digestive system. Trust me, I wish I could spend less time in the bathroom, too" can be enough. Follow up by sending an email with a few links to readings about your disease and your legal rights under the ADA. Sometimes people lash out when they don't fully understand something and helping them learn can squash their difficult behavior. But again, don't share anything you aren't comfortable sharing. (If the coworker is unapproachably toxic, you might want to ask your boss or someone in HR to explain the accommodations on your behalf; I've found that people like this tend to listen to authority figures better than they do colleagues.)

If you're a healthy, able-bodied employee and you see a chronically ill and/or disabled coworker being treated badly, *please* ask what you can do to support them. Use your voice for them. We expect the most marginalized among us to speak up for themselves, but what that really means is that we expect the ones who have the most to lose to put themselves at further risk. In the workplace, healthy, able-bodied folks will continue to wield more power for the foreseeable future.

You might have to take extended time off.

In the United States, the Family and Medical Leave Act (FMLA) lets employees of companies with fifty or more workers take up to twelve weeks off every year for personal or family medical emergencies—but it doesn't require that you get paid during that time (how generous!).[4] It also requires that you've been with the company for twelve months to qualify. On top of FMLA, companies have their own guidelines for unpaid and paid leave; for example, when I needed to take three months off for my long hospitalization in 2015, the company policy gave me 75 percent of my salary for the first part of the leave, then 50 percent, and so on. My company was also flexible on how much time off I needed and protected my job beyond FMLA's twelve weeks. Not every employer will do this, and legally they aren't required to give you your job back after twelve weeks of leave. HR can provide you with your company's specific time off and extended leave policies—when you're chronically ill, these are worth knowing before you accept a position.

If you need longer than twelve weeks away from work, you might want to look into short-term disability. Short-term disability insurance gives you a financial cushion when you can't work for a length of time because of non-job-related illness, injury, or recovery—usually longer than twelve weeks but less than a year. In a handful of states, your employer is legally required to offer a short-term disability insurance plan through the company—but if you live in any other state, it's on you to purchase an annual plan.[5] Most short-term plans aren't going to pay you your full salary—more like 50 or 60 percent—and the payments might not come on the same schedule you're used to. If you need to file for short-term disability, ask your HR department or your

4. "Family and Medical Leave Act," US Department of Labor Wage and Hour Division, last updated October 2019; accessed February 3, 2020, https://www .dol.gov/agencies/whd/fmla.

5. "Comparison of Federal vs. State vs. Private Disability Benefits," Patient Advocate Foundation, last updated July 16, 2019; accessed February 3, 2020, https://www.patientadvocate.org/explore-our-resources/preserving-income -federal-benefits/comparison-of-federal-vs-state-vs-private-disability-benefits/.

doctor's office to help you begin the standard paperwork process. Here's another important thing to know about short-term disability: Unlike FMLA, your job isn't protected. Legally, you can be fired while on short-term disability leave, or your company can give you a different position when you return. But under the ADA, the company has to prove that it has offered all reasonable accommodations before firing you—so there's room to fight if you feel you've been wrongfully terminated or demoted.

If you need a significant length of time away from work, it's time to look into long-term disability insurance (your short-term disability provider should be able to guide you on this, potentially rolling your short-term plan into a long-term one) or Social Security disability, which can be an arduous and emotionally taxing process. The average Social Security disability claim takes three months just to be processed, and you can wait up to two years to go in front of a judge. And then, about 70 percent of initial applicants are denied benefits.[6] Payments are minimal—the average monthly Social Security disability payment as of January 2020 was about $1,200/month.[7] Approval takes court hearings and appeals where you show that you've worked long enough (the official term is *work credits*) to qualify, and that your illness or disability renders you unable to work any longer at any job. I'm not providing this information to dissuade you from applying if it's necessary, I'm just saying: Be ready for a lengthy process.

6. "How to React if Your Social Security Disability Claim or SSI Claim Is Denied," Disability Benefits Center; accessed February 3, 2020, https://www .disabilitybenefitscenter.org/how-to/appeal-social-security-disability-denial.

7. Emily Brandon, "How Much You Will Get from Social Security," *U.S. News and World Reports*, last updated January 21, 2020; accessed February 3, 2020, https://money.usnews.com/money/retirement/social-security/articles/how-much -you-will-get-from-social-security.

If you're unsure about hitting play, it's worth speaking with a Social Security attorney—they can weigh in on whether your claim is likely to be approved and prep you for what to expect. They can also help you find financial assistance while you go through it. Through Social Security disability benefits you'll receive Medicare, which still comes with premiums, deductibles, and co-pays that vary depending on your plan; if you qualify for Supplemental Security Income, which is based on your income level as well as disability or illness, you'll get Medicaid. There's one more thing you should know here—and be warned, it's infuriating. To qualify for SSI, you can't have more than $2,000 in assets as a single person and $3,000 as a married person. This includes cash on hand, checking and savings accounts, stock investments, any cars beyond one, and any homes or properties beyond where you live. Some disabled people avoid getting married—and some avoid even *living with* their partners—because marriage or cohabitation will reduce their benefits.

If you're fired or quit your job, you'll need to get health insurance elsewhere.

If your illness prevents you from working entirely and you don't qualify for disability coverage (and you aren't of an age when you'd be able to receive Medicare), you have three main options, none of which is ideal. First, there's the Consolidated Omnibus Budget Reconciliation Act (COBRA), which lets you stay on your employer-provided health insurance plan for eighteen months (and in some cases, up to thirty-six months) after leaving your job, be it voluntary or involuntary job loss.[8] Here's the thing though: You pay out of pocket for COBRA, and it isn't cheap. Those divine group health insurance plans that take,

---

8. "Continuation of Health Coverage (COBRA)," US Department of Labor; accessed February 3, 2020, https://www.dol.gov/general/topic/health-plans/cobra.

say, $100 or so out of your paycheck thanks to your employer's 70 to 80 percent assistance? Without that help, you're looking at $600 or more on average as an individual for the same plan, and $1,700 if you're supporting a family, plus COBRA charges a 2 percent "administrative fee." You have sixty days to opt in to COBRA from the day your job is terminated.

Under COBRA, there's another law you should know about called the Emergency Medical Treatment and Labor Act, or EMTALA, which applies to all Medicare-participating hospitals. EMTALA aims to provide emergency care to patients regardless of their ability to pay; under the law, the scope of "emergency medical condition" is specific, so do some independent research before going to a hospital and expecting EMTALA coverage. For chronically ill patients whose symptoms have elevated to the point of emergency, EMTALA would require emergency department physicians to stabilize and/or transfer the patient but not to provide ongoing care for the chronic health issue, for example.

When I quit my job at the *Daily Beast* in October 2016, I signed up for COBRA. I originally planned to take a "sabbatical"—a fancy word for "I'm unemployed and have no idea what I'm going to do," but my living expenses made that impossible. COBRA alone cost $1,200/month, but what was the alternative? My bill for a ten-day hospital stay was $100,000 before insurance. By that math, the cost of my longest hospitalization climbed toward seven figures; I shudder to think how much ten years in this body has cost. Depending on where I received my infliximab infusions, the pre-insurance bill could reach $90,000. If I got eight or ten infusions every year, that's $720,000 to $900,000 just to keep me functional. I could pay $1,200/month to keep my insurance plan until signing up for a cheaper and less comprehensive plan through the marketplace, or I could stop my treatment, or go bankrupt. I chose the first option.

COBRA was a nightmare, and not just because it was expensive. My COBRA provider didn't have an online portal—everything was done via snail mail. If my payment got delayed or showed up even a day late, they froze my coverage without notification. At least twice, I showed up to my infusion center to find out I was without insurance coverage and could either pay out of pocket (LOL) or wait until my insurance payment posted. And even then, I'd have to be reapproved for treatment, which could take up to a week. (Why did they have to do this? I still have no idea.) Delaying treatment could—and did, throw me into a flare-up in early 2017, leading to another hospitalization—but all I could do was wait.

Aside from COBRA, there's health insurance through the Affordable Care Act (ACA), which you can sign up for during open enrollment once a year or within thirty days of unemployment through what's called a special enrollment period. (It's how I currently have health insurance.) The ACA is better than nothing, like a wad of gauze is better than an open bullet wound. It's an imperfect system that traps a lot of folks in the "I make too much money to qualify for Medicaid, but all of the ACA plans are too expensive" zone, and ACA premiums—the amount you pay per month—and deductibles—the amount you have to pay before your insurance kicks in—tend to be high, *very* high.[9] Even with an $800/month tax credit, one of the subsidies offered to offset the monthly cost, I still pay $700/month for my health

9. Rachel Nania, "Lower Premiums for Some with 2020 ACA Health Plans," AARP, last updated October 22, 2019; accessed February 3, 2020, https://www.aarp.org/health/health-insurance/info-2019/aca-plans-premium-rates-announced.html.

insurance plan—which isn't all that good, and is sometimes very bad. However, the ACA covers people even with preexisting conditions (Trump tried to take credit for this with a 2020 executive order at the same time his administration was attempting to terminate the ACA as unconstitutional) and won't boot me off my plan for being too expensive, so for that, I'm grateful.

You can sign up through the ACA marketplace online, but if it's your first time, I recommend calling and speaking to a representative because it's a confusing process. They can guide you through the subsidy application process and help you choose the right kind of plan. Have all relevant financial documents ready before you call or apply online and be prepared to estimate your income for *the following year*. Also! Be sure you choose a plan that's accepted by your doctors, rather than picking a plan and finding out later that your doctors are out-of-network. Learn from my mistakes, grasshopper.

Last, there's Medicaid. Medicaid programs vary by state, but basically, they provide health insurance for low-income folks—which you might qualify for if you lost your job and have no income. (There's also the Children's Health Insurance Program, or CHIP, which covers kids in families that have income too high to qualify for Medicaid.) If you live in one of the thirty-eight Medicaid expansion states (that number is as of July 2020), you qualify for the program on household income alone. Be sure to check your state's individual poverty level guidelines; Medicaid usually kicks in at up to 133 percent of the poverty level. If you don't live in an expansion state, income isn't the only factor considered—they'll also weigh family status, disability, and mental health, among other things. (Appallingly, two million low-income adults in non-expansion states don't qualify for Medicaid and also don't qualify for ACA subsidies.) You can apply for Medicaid through the online marketplace just like you would for the ACA (but again, I recommend calling). Medicaid doesn't require you to meet a deductible but still has co-pays, though low, and prescription drug costs. Some states also cap the amount of prescriptions you can fill per month at eight—any more than that and you'll have to get pre-authorization from your doctor, a time-consuming (or rather, time-*wasting*) process that requires your doctor to get the okay from your insurance company before prescribing additional medication.

If you make too much money to qualify for Medicaid but not enough to afford a comprehensive ACA plan, you can get a catastrophic plan that has a lower monthly cost but super high deductible, and it only covers major emergencies.[10] If you're over the age of thirty, you have to qualify for a hardship exemption to get catastrophic coverage; if you're under thirty, you can get it without the exemption. Hardship exemptions cover stuff like homelessness, bankruptcy, significant medical debt, inability to qualify for Medicaid in a non-expansion state, and natural disasters. You can also explore private insurance through a broker—those plans aren't cheap, either—or you can look into a short-term private insurance plan outside of the ACA. These plans can be more affordable per month, but know that they can deny your coverage if you have a preexisting condition (hello, chronic illness) and can cap your benefits—also not good for expensive chronic illness care.

Last, you can join a group plan if you qualify through an organization like the Freelancers Union or the National Association for the Self-Employed, or a medi-share through a religious organization.

---

10. "Catastrophic Health Plans," US Centers for Medicare and Medicaid Services; accessed February 3, 2020, https://www.healthcare.gov/choose-a-plan/catastrophic-health-plans/.

Phew. Won't it be nice when this entire section of the book is irrelevant and we can all access health care without worrying about the cost, insurance or not?

If you plan to quit your job, you need to plan what to say.

If you've decided to leave your job entirely, tell your boss in an email first. Email leaves less room for emotion—if you're like me, you might cry or get flustered when trying to deliver this kind of news in person. Tell them clearly when your last day will be, and, if possible, give at least two weeks' notice. When you've laid out when you're leaving and why (again, share what you're comfortable with; "I'm leaving due to health reasons" is plenty of information), ask to set up an in-person meeting with your boss to discuss the nitty-gritty of your departure. You'll also want to meet with HR to go over your exit paperwork, including your options for health insurance.

You can take action for wrongful termination.

Here's where disclosing your illness in your interview process, or at least early in your employment, becomes important: If an employer fires you and can prove they didn't know about your illness or disability (say you get fired for falling asleep on the job and you haven't told your boss that you have narcolepsy), you may have less power under the guidelines of the ADA. If an employer knows about a chronic illness or disability, they're required to make accommodations—and prove they've *actively* worked with the employee to make those accommodations—before terminating. In a 2014 Federal Court of Appeals ruling,[11] the court spelled this out: "If an employee tells his employer that he has a disability, the employer then knows of the disability, and the ADA's further requirements bind the employer." (I've

---

11. Spurling v. C&M Fine Pack, Inc. (7th Cir. 2014).

added more information in Appendix VIII about how to proceed if you think you've been wrongfully terminated.)

The first question we ask anyone we meet, after exchanging names, is "What do you do?" Then we make snap judgments—untrue ones, usually—based on the answer: Accountants are boring but safe. Teachers are selfless but poor. Doctors are arrogant but respectable. Lawyers are smart but sleazy. Actors are sexy but fickle. Writers are creative but mad (maybe this one is true). The answer to "What do you do?" tells us stuff we place value on: Working long hours must mean you're dedicated; making a lot of money must mean you're smart; having a certain title must mean you're successful. None of this is accurate, of course, but all of us employ these conclusions to categorize people. When the answer is "I'm unable to work anymore," the judgment is "lazy, unmotivated, mediocre." Our identities get tangled up in what we do for a living, and when that changes or ends due to chronic illness, it makes us feel as if we don't know who we are or what we offer to the world. We become fearful of how others think of us.

It's easy enough to figure out how to take a leave of absence or how to sign up for COBRA, but it isn't easy redefining your identity when it's been built around what you do for a living. It's heartbreaking to be ambitious and have chronic illness get in the way of your goals and dreams. It isn't something you just get over; in the face of lifelong illness, you have to dig in and redefine what success means to you. You must remind yourself that you're a human being worthy of love and respect—whether you have a career or not. Like Julie Andrews when she lost her voice, you have to find a new way to do what gives you meaning.

Though I didn't give up my career entirely, I still get lost wondering what it would look like had I never gotten sick. Illness has taught me a lot, but it hasn't fully tamed my ego, ever-hungry for power and distinction and Twitter followers. What has helped, though, is to remember why I became a journalist in the first place: because I love writing and reading and telling stories. Senior year of high school, an economics class required me to write a paper about my dream career; I chose journalism. I was unaware then of the ins and outs of the media industry or how brutal it could be, but I knew journalists told stories for a living and that sounded better than any other job I could think of. Greg Kot, the *Chicago Tribune*'s longtime music critic, agreed to an interview for that paper and I can still recall the rush of speaking to someone I wanted to be like. Today, I don't have a fancy title or a desk at a prestigious publication. I'm not exactly a journalist anymore, not in the way I'd planned to be, but I'm still telling stories. I like to think seventeen-year-old me would be proud, even if things turned out different than I thought they would.

CHAPTER 15

Very, Very Not *Normal*

I am writing to you from the Perlmutter Cancer Center at NYU Langone. It's on the eighth floor of the tallest building around here, in a South Brooklyn neighborhood called Midwood. To my left is a bright yellow bin that says "NON RCRA HAZ-ARDOUS WASTE FOR INCINERATION EMPTY CHE-MOTHERAPY IV BAGS." To my right, the machine I'm hooked up to via IV beeps as it dispenses medication over a two-hour session. Sitting in front of me is the nurses' station, with a keyboard, monitor, and TV that I've never attempted to turn on. I measure time in six-week intervals, planning life around when I'm due to come here, when the medication will be at its highest level, and when I'll begin to feel it wearing off.

The rooms here are divided by heavy curtains, and I can hear *The Price Is Right* playing from the TV in the room next to mine. The chairs are cushiony leather things with a footrest and a reclining back. My feet are tucked under me and I'm curled up in a white waffle-weave blanket that just came out of a warmer. Greg is sitting across from me doing his law school reading.

I've learned to like it here in this mundane health center. It's predictable and I like predictability: check in, get wristband, be called back, get weighed, pee in cup, go to designated numbered room, wait for nurse to start IV (fingers crossed it takes a single poke), swallow two Tylenol pills, get IV Benadryl, wait for pharmacy to mix infliximab, feel IV Benadryl kick in (*whoaaaaa*), do nurse's check and codes, start infusion. Then wait some more. Every infusion, I take a photo of whichever hand has the IV giving a "thumbs-up," and I send the photo to Mom to signal that all is well. I never miss an appointment. If infliximab keeps working, I'll be coming here—or somewhere like it—for the rest of my life. Sometimes people ask, "How long will you need medication?" The answer is forever, so long as I can access it. If I don't develop antibodies to infliximab, I'll be on it *forever*. And if I do develop antibodies, I'll switch to another biologic, all of which are named with some gobbledygook ending in *mab*. But no matter which drugs I switch to, the answer remains *forever*, which isn't what people like to hear. Humans prefer to categorize illness: Either you're cured or you're not. But illnesses like mine can be managed, not cured, and that shakes our understanding of what it means to be sick or well. There's a vast in-between where people like me exist.

Perlmutter is my third infusion center. I've been coming here for three years now, and it's good because Doc's office is one floor below. Next to Doc's office is the oncologist who oversees my treatment since it's technically chemotherapy. And I know the nurses here well, too. I inquire about their kids and their graduate study programs. They ask how this book is coming along and, when Greg's not with me, how he's handling law school. My favorite nurse knows where my one good vein is, marked by an old, round hospital scar just above my wrist, so she gets my IV started in one try—quite a feat with my skinny, rolling, scarred veins. We talk about our lives outside of work and illness, and I look forward to seeing her like I would a friend.

Before I started coming here, insurance assigned me to two other infusion centers, each one a little different. At Columbia's Cancer Center in Washington Heights, the wait was long and the infusion longer—a four-hour drip, slow to avoid a reaction. Some days I'd be there for seven or eight hours from start to finish. But I had a real room, with walls, and a friendly lady with a snack cart came around offering fruit cups, potato chips, and juice boxes. The second was a privately owned oncology center on Fourth Avenue in Park Slope. The wait and infusion were long there, too, and there was no privacy—everyone got treatment in a circle around the perimeter of the room, like a depressing campfire. Once, while getting my infusion there, I watched a young woman walk from the entrance doors to the nurses' desk and tell them that her mother wouldn't be coming to her chemotherapy appointment. Through tears, she told the nurses that her mom had died. They all cried together and hugged. I wondered how many patients these nurses had lost and if it ever got easier.

I'm lucky, see. Though complications of Crohn's disease can and do kill people, as long as my disease stays managed as it is now, and as long as I don't get a secondary infection, I can live just as long as I would were I healthy. My illness isn't terminal. Still, I sometimes feel very *un*lucky. I have wished for finality, for escape, for an end to my illness—even if that meant death. Is dying better than living life with incurable illness? The answer is, for me, no. But it took a long time for me to decide that my life *is* still worth living, even more so, with forever sickness. And it's completely normal to question it, as I've discovered in my support groups and via conversations with other chronically ill people. "I don't think I can live like this anymore" remains a common sentiment—and an understandable one. Some people even expressed jealousy of folks with terminal illnesses: "At least there's an ending." No one wants to *not* live, but they do want to be free from pain and fear.

When I was at my lowest—wondering if I would die from *C. diff,* wading through panic attacks, languishing in Methodist for weeks, getting an *E. coli* infection—I wish someone would have told me that on the other side of this sort of terrible ache comes *joy,* like the pressing of ashes into diamond. True, immense joy that only came from being in the trenches. Before my diagnosis, gratitude was reserved for big, mostly selfish moments: graduations, job offers, promotions, getting my writing published. After life-threatening illness and extended hospital stays, something shifted. I was grateful to be alive, sure, but it was more than that. I sensed the sun on my skin as I had thousands of times before but now noticed and appreciated its warmth. I felt connected to strangers when I walked through my neighborhood, a little farther each day as I got stronger. I started seeking out and listening to music again—something that made me too sad after Dad died. Instead of treating people with resentment or comparison, I turned to empathy. My pain was different from their pain, but that didn't make it any more valuable. I didn't come out of the hospital wishing I'd spent more hours at work or fought harder for a promotion. I wished that I'd told my parents all the complicated ways I loved them, and Kaetlyn how proud I was of her. I wished I'd taken better care of my brain and my heart, learning more and reading more. I wished I'd belly laughed without hesitation, been sillier, not taken it all so seriously.

No doubt there's a mania that occurs when you get out of the hospital after being uncertain you would, and that contributed to some of my feelings. Everything seemed brighter and louder and tasted better. *Holy shit, I'm alive! I can turn on the tap and get hot water—WOW! I can order the best food I've ever tasted right from my phone—AMAZING! I'm surrounded by stunning people and plants and animals—SHAZAM!* But as that *holy shit-ness* faded, I still held on to gratitude and the joy it brought because it made me better, stronger. It turned angrily hating myself and my circumstances into an act of observing and thanking.

This isn't to say practicing gratitude is easy or comes naturally—it takes constant awareness and the courage to keep trying. My online friend, the writer Jonny Sun, wrote, "I think people who ridicule positivity think positivity is easy. Don't shut out the bad. Take it in and in the face of it, choose to do good." The same goes for optimism and compassion. It's radical to choose gratitude when you've been dealt a shitty hand. It's a big *fuck you* to the forces that keep you feeling defeated. (On the other hand, it's simple to choose gratitude when all your needs are met, like safety, sustained health, food, shelter, money, work, and access to health care. I call this "influencer gratitude" or "hashtag gratitude.") And being thankful doesn't mean you're always happy—gratitude and unhappiness can coexist, as they often do for me. Allowing sadness, sitting with that discomfort and exploring where it comes from, *feeling it all*, is what paves the road for unfettered joy. Like Claire Bidwell Smith told me: "You can feel sad and create a meaningful, joyful life."

Through self-reflection, therapy, and a commitment to empathy, I realized that my pain wasn't big or small, it just *was*. Individual pain feels big—giant, even—because it's all we know in our brains and bodies. It's our only perspective. It's *ours*. The one hundred pounds in your invisible buckets feel very heavy even when your neighbor is carrying two hundred pounds. As I connected with chronically ill folks, I understood that my pain was never better or worse than anyone else's. Weighing my struggles against those of others wasn't helpful to me or to them. Think about it: If a friend came to you in pain, would you tell them that other people have it worse and that their pain isn't valid? If you did, you'd be a lousy friend—so why do you speak to yourself in such a way? (Awareness of your privilege in how you deal with pain *is* important, though. A thin, white, cis woman like me is going to navigate the health-care system more easily than most, and that ease in itself is going to decrease my mental and physical pain.)

Instead of playing the who-has-it-better-or-worse game like I did at the start of my illness, I ask for support when I need it and give support when I can. Junior year of college, right after Dad died, I took an intro-level class about Buddhism. I was trying to feel close to him, making some sense of his death by exploring the closest thing to religion he'd practiced. The professor said something that's stuck with me all these years: "It is our job to give without asking why." If a fellow chronically ill person comes to me for support, it is my job to help them if I can, however I can, without comparing our pain. When a *healthy* person comes to me for support, it is my job to help them without comparison, too. And when I give freely, I feel joy. I know now that pain—physical and emotional—is only one part of me and I don't have to let it be the loudest.

As much as I've learned, it's still difficult at times to overcome the fear of an uncertain future. I'm in remission now, but that could change at any moment if my body decides to reject my medication. I could end up with *C. diff* again or catch any other infection (hello, COVID) waiting to prey on my lousy immune system. This kind of uncertainty used to cause panic, and though I can still sometimes feel it rising through my chest, I've learned how to manage it. I call these "my soothers." Do these come naturally to me? No. My instinct is to stand in front of the mirror and shred my face bloody, then spend two weeks slathering it in creams and oils until it heals, only to do it all over again. But I know that won't make me feel better in the long run, so I've established a bunch of (better) tricks to use in place of self-mutilation.

First, I tell myself that it's okay to be scared. It's normal. I let the feeling move through me instead of trying to bury it, because I know that if I do repress it, it will fight to break out in the form of a panic attack. I take deep breaths. I go for a walk with my dogs. I take a hot shower or a long bath. I talk to Greg. I call Kaetlyn. I look at funny memes and send them to my friends. I "window-shop" online, adding stuff to a cart that I'll never buy. I remind myself that I've made it this far, and that I don't need to have control over every single thing. I also do this thought exercise that a friend taught me; it's a little *woo-woo*, but bear with me:

We all carry around versions of ourselves—different ages, circumstances. When we're scared and out of control in the present, we must take a moment to think about where and *when* that feeling is coming from. Then "show" that version of yourself that *you are safe now.* Show the ten-year-old in a violent home that they're safe. Show the twenty-five-year-old in the hospital that they're home. Show the fourteen-year-old with an eating disorder that they have better coping mechanisms. Get it? It's a simple exercise, but for me, it's been powerful. I used to dream, sometimes weekly during sleep, about scooping my childhood self up and running away, somewhere. Anywhere. This exercise is sort of a coordinated version of that dream.

I also try to avoid catastrophizing. *I have a chronic illness and it's going to flare up. I know this, and I can take steps to manage it. If it gets really bad, well, I've been through it before and came out the other side. I have treatment options left should infliximab fail, and I have doctors I trust to help me through my decisions.* I'm fortunate to be sick *now*, when living well with IBD is possible thanks to new medication, well-funded research, and finessed surgical procedures. Even fifty years ago, a Crohn's diagnosis usually meant a life of pain followed by a steady decline into death via infection, blockage, or some other complication.

And though I'm lucky to be on the right IBD medication, it's not the only factor that's contributed to my current run of good health. I've actively made big and small life changes, too. I cut gluten out of my diet to control the symptoms of celiac disease. I stopped eating out much—too many factors to worry about—and I cook at home with mostly fresh ingredients. I find a lot of satisfaction in preparing food for myself and for Greg, whose excited reactions to whatever I serve for dinner make it worth it each time. ("This is the best thing I've ever eaten!" he says every time.) Plus, I'm pretty good at it, thanks in part to many years of cooking with Mom out of necessity—we could do a lot with rice and government-issued cheese. I take an antidepressant before bed, without fail, every night. I get my medication refilled on time and I see my psychiatrist as needed, though not as often as I should or would like to, due to cost. I have a good dermatologist who, along with my psychiatrist, helped me stop coping with anxiety by picking my skin. I don't drink alcohol anymore, save a sip of wine at a special occasion once or twice a year, because the physical and mental effects weren't benefiting me, and because I want to support Kaetlyn in her sobriety (three years and counting; I'm so proud of you, Sis). I work from home and make my own schedule. I never miss an infliximab infusion. I don't wait until a crisis to see Doc. I'm proud of myself for being proactive, when my instincts are to freeze and pretend difficult stuff isn't happening. I really, truly care about and prioritize the well-being of my body and mind. Who would have thought? (Not me!)

Additionally, I've gained professional direction from chronic illness through my writing. The first time I wrote publicly about being sick forever was at the end of 2013, in an essay about being diagnosed with IBD and the experience of my first fecal transplant. I was terrified. *Everyone is going to label me as "that sick girl." I will never work again. People will think I'm disgusting. This will come up every time someone Googles me. I am embarrassing myself and my family.* But when the piece was published, I was met with astounding support. Hundreds of chronically ill folks emailed or sent me messages on social media, relaying stories similar to and different from my own, but all with a common message: "What you wrote made me feel seen." Friends and acquaintances told me they better understood what I'd been through. "I had no idea," some of them said. It felt good. I kept writing, and people from all over the world kept reaching out to me with their own stories. I'd been so scared to share this huge, defining part of my life for fear of negative judgment, but I was met with the opposite: acceptance. Even Mom, who I'm always so afraid to hurt when I write about the hard stuff, has never stood in my way or made me feel as though I have limits on what I can and can't share. "I'm committed to your truth," she said. What a gift.

When I wrote the first three-quarters of this chapter, reflecting on what I've gained from my experiences thus far, COVID-19 was still a mysterious illness seemingly contained to the city of Wuhan, China, and news about the novel respiratory disease didn't make it above the newspaper fold. But by March 2020, it was an entirely different world. My life was more "normal" than it ever had been before—my health remained steady, my relationship strong, my family stable—and yet just beyond me, nothing was normal. People were rightly afraid, anxious, and suffering. Jobs were lost en masse and, with them, health insurance. Our health-care workers—three out of four of whom are women—went without proper masks and gowns and gloves (meanwhile, militarized police were armed to the teeth against Black Lives Matter crowds). Families couldn't gather to mourn their dead, and morgues and funeral homes in the hardest-hit cities ran out of space. Scariest of all, the most anti-science president to ever hold the office was expected to lead us through it—a man who refused to wear a mask in public (save for once during a visit to Walter Reed Medical Center, when 135,000 Americans were already dead from the virus), who called for less virus testing to bolster his campaign, who muzzled our country's leading scientists, and who, even before that, pulled out of the Paris Agreement and said windmills cause cancer, vaccines are linked to autism, and hurricanes can be stopped with nuclear weapons. His COVID response was *Do next to nothing, then pretend it's over.* That he was the one in charge during the worst pandemic of our lifetime would be darkly funny if it wasn't so damn terrifying.

The COVID-19 pandemic revealed all the cracks in our health-care and social systems; even the slightest stress resulted in widespread failure for the most vulnerable. (Can a country that doesn't readily provide health care to its citizens ever truly be prepared for a pandemic? I'd argue no.) Americans have been trained in individualism since birth and, under the weight of a pandemic, were expected to care about our communities. *Imagine that! Thinking of others before ourselves!* Coronavirus wasn't a great equalizer, as politicians liked to say. It hurt and killed the people already most at risk in an unjust system. And as we learn more about the long-term health effects of the illness among a group dubbed "long haulers," I can't stop thinking: This has created a whole new population of chronically ill people, and no one in power seems to care.

Trump's own COVID diagnosis was perhaps the best illustration of these inequalities. After testing positive for the virus in early October, he was airlifted from his home to a private hospital suite and given around-the-clock care with access to costly experimental treatments, with no fear of the bill. When he was discharged back to the White House, Trump's first act was to defiantly remove his mask for a photo op, seemingly to display his masculinity or toughness (things that do not, in fact, conflate with one's ability to recover from illness; access to quality care, on the other hand, *does*). And not once, during or after his hospitalization, did Trump express sympathy or concern for the hundreds of thousands of Americans who died not just from COVID, but from his administration's negligence. If the virus mattered at all to Trump, it was because it happened to *him*.

(I should note here that the final version of this book is being sent to print before I know the outcome of the presidential election. As I write this, I do not know who wins in 2020. What I do know is that there won't be a landslide repudiation of Trump, no movie ending where the masses rise up to cast him out. In the thick of a pandemic that kills 1,000 people a day, half of voters will still pick the very bad guy because he helps them maintain a mental hierarchy where they're "better" because they're white or male or Christian or able-bodied or whatever. Without that hierarchy, their whole understanding of the world and their place in it crumbles and, well, that wouldn't feel very nice, would it? Our country is built on all kinds of cruelty, and that's how many of its citizens—chiefly its white citizens—survive and thrive. Election results can't change that.)

My beloved home, New York City, was early on the hardest-hit metropolitan area in the country. At the start of the outbreak, available tracking showed my neighborhood to be a red zone (meaning among those being tested for COVID-19, the highest percentages were testing positive). I've been social distancing and self-quarantining as needed since 2012, and I already work from home. I'm in the habit of hand washing and mask wearing. I don't go to bars. Rarely, I venture into a restaurant. It was a weird relief to have others finally follow suit. So I wasn't all that concerned about getting COVID-19 since I was taking every precaution not to. I worried more that my Crohn's symptoms would flare up and I'd need to go to a hospital, where the viral risk would be too great and the system too overwhelmed.

Still, with all these concerns, I wasn't sure if we should leave. I've dedicated ten years of my life to being sick in New York, even when I knew it would be easier anywhere else. We were sheltering in place before it was mandated, but Greg was terrified that simply running to the grocery store would bring the virus home to me. If I caught COVID-19, I could end up incredibly sick and likely hospitalized. Staying here felt like tempting fate.

Greg became adamant: "It isn't safe for you to be here. We need to go *now*. Not in three days. Now." Greg is the real New Yorker in our relationship, not me. He was born in New York, as was his mother before him and his first-generation grandparents before her. He stayed through 9/11, more dedicated to the city than ever, when his apartment window overlooked the Twin Towers. "Dude, look outside," his neighbor said on the phone when he called Greg that clear September morning. "The world is ending." When Greg said we had to leave, I knew it was serious.

I guess this is the part of the book where I tell you more about Greg. Admittedly, I'm afraid to even write about my marriage because it's *now*, and most of the memoir in this book covers *then*. It's always been easier for me to write about the past because I can't change it, but I'm actively contributing to the present and that is scary to put on a page.

There's this popular quote from John Green's YA novel *The Fault in Our Stars* (which I have, admittedly, never read) that says, "I fell in love the way you fall asleep: slowly, and then all at once." I fell in love with Greg in the completely opposite way—*immediately*—just hoping he'd live up to the life I'd created for us before we'd even finished shaking hands. It's no hyperbole: I knew I was going to marry Greg within fifteen seconds of meeting him. Thankfully, he felt the same or else it would've gotten weird fast.

When we met by chance that June week, the same week I moved out of my shared apartment with Jimmy, I was still wearing my engagement ring out of habit. I wondered what people would think about me "moving on" so quickly, but I didn't really care. Maybe Greg was the Fates' gift for finally doing something right in canceling my wedding with Jimmy; not fake right, for appearances. But right for myself, right for *real*. A force greater than me was like, "Oh, I see you're finally getting it. Here, have an angel!"

We never would have met had I not been courageous enough to call off the wedding, had my friend not taken me out for breakup sushi and a good cry session before dragging me to "some illegal traveling speakeasy" after dinner. I hate bars and avoid them. Even when I still drank alcohol, I was always trying to "step outside for a phone call" after dinner and sneak into a cab before anyone could convince me to go out on the town. I didn't do "after hours" or even "regular hours." But it was a perfect June night when I met Greg—just humid enough to make

226 | WHAT DOESN'T KILL YOU

your skin glow—and I wasn't ready to go home and be alone, so I agreed. Five months later, Greg asked me to marry him with a $200 ring in the parking lot of the Queens Center Mall. Fifteen months after that, we got married at City Hall in Manhattan with Kaetlyn and Zoe as our witnesses. It was Zoe's fourteenth birthday. We ate gluten-free chocolate cake after the ceremony and then went out for steaks. It was perfect.

From the start, Greg has given me the gift of feeling safe. He's predictable—I mean that in the best way—and reliable. If he says he's going to do something, he does it. He's slow to anger and infinitely gentle. Animals and babies are drawn to him. He saves his pizza crusts to give to our dogs and calls them "pizza bones." He plays this game where he tries to make customer service agents' days brighter by being incessantly nice to them on the phone. A New York Italian American, Greg says words like "muhtzahrell," "pro-shoot," "bisgott," and "baciagaloop," but without any stereotyped mafioso chauvinism. He always smells like a little kid after recess—sweat and grass and fresh air. He makes me laugh by putting on music and flailing around akin to one of those inflatable car dealership noodles, or singing songs in a voice that sounds like Frank Sinatra as a Muppet. He comes with me to doctor's appointments and infusions, not because I need him to but because he wants to—even though he has to step out of the room when I get an IV; the "circulatory system on the outside" freaks him out, he says.

But like all my favorite people, Greg is not without darkness. He's been chronically depressed since adolescence and spent years searching for the right combination of treatment and medication—Lexapro, Wellbutrin, Lamictal, Ritalin, Ativan, propranolol, ketamine, genetic testing, brain scans, cognitive behavioral therapy, hypnotherapy, eye movement desensitization and reprocessing. At his lowest, he spent weeks-long stretches in bed, suffocated by an invisible, paralyzing darkness. For years, he visualized how he'd kill himself and, when the suicidal ideation became all-consuming, he checked himself into a psychiatric hospital for two weeks. Since then, Greg has been in regular therapy and found an SSRI that works. As a kid, he wanted to be a homemaker like his mom. But he ended up being a successful clothing designer instead, making, among other things, David Bowie's final tour wardrobe, which now lives in the Rock and Roll Hall of Fame. When he became disillusioned with the fashion industry, at age forty-five, he took the LSAT and enrolled in law school with a focus on public service. Depression is more of a memory than a daily visitor. My biggest fear is that Greg will become depressed again, so depressed that even I can't reach him. His biggest fear is that my medication will stop working or that I'll get some kind of deadly infection. How right that we ended up together.

People like to say, "Marriage is supposed to be hard!" but I've found it to be the exact opposite. *Everything else* is hard, but marriage? Marriage is my safe place. Greg can fix things, literally and metaphorically, that I can't. He knows how to build stuff from scrap wood, he can start a fire without a match, and though he's a pacifist to his core, he can throw a killer right hook. (I know because I've seen his score on the Coney Island punch machine: 900.) He's strong in a sinewy kind of way, compact and tightly wound and strong-jawed. He's levelheaded and fair and he offers me grace over anger, even when I'm being a real asshole. I've often joked that he's the person I want on my end of the world team (and since, as I write this, reality's looking pretty apocalyptic, I'm in the best possible place).

In 2018, Greg's parents built a homestead on a remote chunk of 130 acres in western North Carolina, on mountainous land that belonged to the Cherokee and Catawba before it was stolen by the English and Scotch Irish. Now it's a vacation house for my in-laws and for us a few months out of the year, sitting empty during the worst of New York's outbreak. With encouragement from my doctors, we threw some clothes and snacks in a bag, packed up the dogs, and drove ten hours south through the lush, rolling emerald of the Virginias. I wasn't sure if we were doing the right thing; to me, it felt like fleeing, just like those rich folks of yesteryear. There were media stories about wealthy people deserting the city for the Hamptons, but more quietly among my chronically ill friends and support circles, people left for their parents' homes in some place you've never heard of. I can count a dozen more who, between March and August 2020, moved out of New York City for good, as life there was no longer doable with underlying disease and the risk of COVID. I came to this conclusion: When you're chronically ill in a pandemic, you do what you need to do to stay alive.

We spent one hundred days in North Carolina, going nowhere and seeing no one except other grocery store patrons. Six weeks into sheltering in place, my insurance company had to grant permission for me to get an infusion at the nearby center. Seems like an easy enough request, right? Here's what I had to do to get my medication out of state: Call my insurance company. Speak to two representatives who tell me that I absolutely cannot get my infusion outside of New York State, and that they aren't making any concessions even though NYC is a COVID-19 hotbed. Beg. Plead. Tell them it's not safe for me to be in New York. Feel hot tears coming down my cheeks. Try not to get angry at these customer service reps who I know don't make the rules. Tweet at insurance company. Insurance company sees I have blue Twitter checkmark and that tweet is getting lots of negative attention.

Insurance company asks me to DM them my phone number, saying someone will call me. Hours pass—then days. No one calls. DM insurance company. Nothing. Tweet at insurance company, since that seems to be the only way to get a response. Insurance company says someone will call me. Someone calls me. They say I can get my medication out of state no problem: "Go to any CVS." I explain that it's an infusion. They say I need prior authorization, which means Doc has to prove that I need the medication I've taken for half a decade. I ask: Do I need authorization from my doctor in New York, or from the doctor (whom I haven't seen yet) here in North Carolina? They aren't sure. They will call me back in ten minutes. Twenty minutes pass. Thirty. Email Doc's office to get prior authorization in motion. Tell the office administrator to be thorough and specific. Call nearby infusion center to be sure they provide infliximab infusions. Set up appointment to see doctor at new infusion center. Know that after all this, insurance company could still deny treatment. Wait. Get automated call. "Your doctor's pre-authorization has been denied." Tweet. Get other people to tweet. Cry some more. Talk to Mom. "I emailed Senator Schumer's office!" she says. Talk to Kaetlyn. "My friends are signing up for Twitter to help you!" she says. DM insurance company, again. No response. Go to bed. Wake up. Get phone call from insurance company. "Did you switch medication?" Remember that insurance company made me switch to biosimilar last November. Tell them technically yes, I switched to infliximab-*abda* because you made me, even though my doctor appealed to keep me on brand-name infliximab. "We'll call you back." Wait. Email NYC's public advocate office. Wait more. Wonder how I can move to Canada. Read hundreds of tweets from people I know and people I don't telling insurance company to do the right thing. Be glad for the support but feel embarrassed that this is what it's come to and angry on behalf of people who can't wage this kind of public campaign. Get automated call. "Your doctor's pre-authorization has been approved." Call insurance company. "Is the approval for out of state?" I ask. They aren't sure. They'll call me back. More hours pass. Insurance company calls. "We have good news: Your out-of-state infusion has been approved." Notice I haven't taken a deep breath in three days. I should feel celebratory, but I'm just tired. *Why does it have to be this hard?* The day before I'm due for treatment, the infusion center calls and says I'm not approved after all. They cancel my appointment. I call the insurance company and leave a message. No call back. I call the infusion center to find out more. They're closed. I call the next day. They're at lunch. I call insurance company again and leave a message. Wait. What an American problem, to be faced with flinging myself back into a virus hot zone because my health insurance company says I have to.

Two weeks delayed from my six-week schedule, I was finally able to get my medication. The insurance coordinator was on the phone with my provider as my appointment began—so even as I sat, masked and gloved, next to the machine that would hold the bag of infliximab-abda, I was unsure if I'd be able to receive it. After two painstaking hours, the head doctor got on the phone to yell at the insurance provider: "This woman needs this medicine. What is wrong with you?!" A nurse started my IV moments later. When I left, I ordered flowers to thank the staff for their weeks of work helping me. I had one more infusion there before my insurance company wouldn't approve further treatment—and by then, it was safer in New York than North Carolina where COVID was concerned. (And I cried tears of joy when I finally saw the NYC skyline, knowing I'd be home soon in the greatest city in the world.) When I got back to Brooklyn, a letter from the insurance company was waiting for me: "This is a notice that we're raising your monthly premium by 22 percent." *I am so tired.*

But in a backward way, I was well prepared for this sort of maddening problem. I was familiar with challenging my health insurance company on almost every decision they make; had I not been sick for so many years, I wouldn't have known how to fight them (though I'm still in awe at the callousness of making me work this hard for such a simple request during a goddamn pandemic).

Even if I was better prepared for a pandemic than most, I still woke up every morning in the spring and into the summer of 2020 with a thick gnawing of anxiety. It felt like stage fright, but with no outlet. Like hunger, but with no fill. For ten glorious seconds each morning before my consciousness came online, I didn't remember where or who I was. And then, like a cartoon piano falling on my head, The Dread kicked in. I thought about asking my psychiatrist for benzos. *No, maybe I'll smoke a little pot instead.* Should I try drinking a glass of wine? *I know that won't help.* A walk in the woods? A Netflix escape binge? A hot shower? Cuddling the dogs? I've tried all the things—all my "soothers." Some distracted me for a few moments. And bit by bit, my brain caught up to my body. My belly filled with painful gas. Day and night, it felt like someone was playing a drum in my rectum. The skin around my butthole tore, fissured by inflammation. The delay of my medication combined with stress I couldn't seem to escape, and my disease became active for the first time in three years. When I went to the bathroom the day before turning in this book's manuscript to my publisher, there was blood on the toilet paper. My body never lets me forget that I'll always be sick.

So, sure, the fear and isolation and uncertainty of living through a pandemic offer some insight into what it's like to live with chronic illness. But if you're able-bodied, then there's no way you could entirely understand—and I wouldn't wish for you to, as it would require you to become sick forever.

What you can do, though, is translate those inklings of understanding into empathy; I don't mean simply imagining how chronically ill people move through the world, I mean *action*. I saw this on a graffiti sticker in my Brooklyn neighborhood, a quote by prison abolitionist Mariame Kaba: *Let this radicalize you*. Empathy is more than putting yourself in someone else's shoes; it's using your power to fight for changes that don't directly benefit you. It's more than understanding why another person feels the way they do; it's learning about the systems (or lack of) that contribute to their emotions and behaviors, then figuring out how you can help build or dismantle and rebuild those systems. What good is putting yourself in someone else's shoes if you're going to stand immobile in them, instead of figuring out how to run? Maybe you rarely have to consider your health insurance, or think about what it means to exist in a politicized body, or save up a reserve for health emergencies. Your world is not *the* world. You must care even when—especially when—issues aren't immediately yours. Act on your empathy however you can: Educate yourself and others about chronic illness and our inequitable health-care system, actively fight against ableism, expand the voices and information you consume, research your legislators' views and records on public health and then become a thorn in their sides, volunteer at a hospital or with a political campaign, canvass, phone bank, vote, march, show up for your town hall meetings, mobilize, donate to mutual aid funds. Do two of these things. Do three. Do all of them. And do them every day, not just every four years when the pressure of an election moves you. Do *something* every single day that shows you not only care, but that you're working toward a better, more just world. Empathy is love, and love is action.

CHAPTER 16

Seven Secrets

Though I write publicly about chronic illness, there are still things I'm afraid to say to those closest to me. It's daunting to have strangers read the most intimate details of my life, but it's even scarier to let the people closest to me in on them. I'd rather play to a stadium than a living room. And despite what the writing of a memoir signals, I don't love to talk about myself IRL; the page makes me appear much braver than I am. But despite the fear, I keep sharing my stories through writing because that's how humans connect and stay alive. Stories gift us empathy. They make us strong. They offer perspective. As James Baldwin wrote, "You think your pain and your heartbreak are unprecedented in the history of the world, but then you read." And, selfishly perhaps, writing helps me regain some of the power that's been lost to my illness. Writing is a way for me to *not* disappear. But it isn't easy, even after all these years. When I pitched this book, one publisher rejected it because "poop stuff is too hard to read about." That comment made my cheeks burn with embarrassment, as though there was something wrong with writing the truth about my body. (Little did that publisher know, doing things because someone told me I couldn't or shouldn't is my

234 | WHAT DOESN'T KILL YOU

brand. Kaetlyn likes to tease that anything I've ever achieved is out of sheer spite.)

But still, I harbor secrets about my illness. I keep them partly to shelter my loved ones and partly to protect myself. I don't want my family to worry or think they need to jump on a plane every time I have a flare-up. I don't want Greg to see me as a burden. What I crave is to wake up each day independent and capable, rejecting the notion that illness alone defines me. And so, I keep secrets— some big, some small. At times, the only place I feel safe sharing is in my support groups, where I know that those around me are carrying similar fears and shame. I'm tired. We're tired. Dread and embarrassment are a heavy load, and it only gets heavier with time, leading to guilt, blame, resentment, and self-loathing. Secrets don't fight any of those feelings—only honesty can do that.

So here I've gathered what I believe are seven of the most pressing—or most commonly discussed, perhaps—secrets chronically ill folks keep; seven secrets that our loved ones should know. I came up with this list from living in a forever-sick body, but also through talking to chronically ill friends, support group members, and online connections. My hope is that this chapter will begin conversations among chronically ill people and those close to them, and that those discussions will be a first step toward lightening the burden chronically ill folks carry. As the old Alcoholics Anonymous saying goes, "You're only as sick as your secrets."

Secret #1: We're sick (no pun intended) of unsolicited advice.

Our friends and families want to be supportive. They want to feel useful, to take an active role in our health. But chronic illness is just that—chronic, meaning a cure doesn't exist yet. Yoga, essential oils, aloe juice, apple cider vinegar, fad diets, meditation, prayer, chiropractors, prebiotics, probiotics, and acupuncture aren't going to magically stop an illness that doctors, researchers, and other scientific minds can't yet crack. Simplifying wellness into "drink more water" or "just do yoga" abandons all the complexity of what makes up health: an array of genetic, environmental, and social issues. Among ourselves, chronically ill people joke about how rich we'd be if we had a nickel for every time someone recommended Pilates or told us to shove rose quartz up our butts. In one of my support groups, we laughed about not only the things people have told us to do to cure IBD but also the *wild* things we've been told caused it: karma, aliens, lack of faith, lack of prayer, weakness of character, STDs, vaccines, eating junk food, eating meat, not eating meat, negative energy, godly punishment, whatever your mother ate while pregnant, low self-esteem. (Remember that stuff from three chapters ago about sickness and godlessness in old-time society? Still alive and kicking!) A lot of people mistake IBD for IBS, or think the ulceration caused by IBD is the same as something like a peptic ulcer (it's not). And celiac disease, an immune response to gluten that causes permanent intestinal damage, gets lumped in with fad diets.

Chronically ill people are told all the time that we just need to "boost" our immune systems. Take this vitamin, drink this elixir, eat this superfood! *The cure is just there, you see? On the shelf.* It's comforting to think that a solution exists no farther than the drugstore. But the immune system doesn't need to be boosted at all; in fact, when the immune system does overreact, it can cause deadly allergic reactions, autoimmune diseases that attack healthy tissue (like Crohn's), and cytokine storms (a type of which causes the lungs to fill with overly aggressive immune cells, like we're seeing in COVID-19 patients). The immune system is like a ballet, delicately balanced but powerful; when the routine goes as practiced, it appears effortless. But one overextension of a leg and the whole move goes wrong.

See, the immune system is composed of three parts: barriers, like skin; the innate immune responses you're born with, like how your body responds to a cold with a fever and snotty nose; and the adaptive responses your immune system learns over your lifetime, such as immunity to chicken pox either through virus or vaccine. Your body's inflammatory response is a good thing—in the case of a cold or flu—but becomes harmful when it starts attacking healthy cells. And there's absolutely no scientific proof that most fad "inflammation fighter" products do much at all for the immune system. (Like I said before: Some inflammation is good! That's how your body is supposed to respond. If the label on a bottle of juice or non-FDA-accepted supplement says "Reduces inflammation," you can guess it's probably fraud.) Science points to just two things that *do* help the functionality of the immune system: getting plenty of sleep and reducing stress.

Some of the stuff people tend to recommend is fine in conjunction with regular medical treatment. If praying helps your mental well-being or lavender oil is part of your bedtime routine, that's great. But the underlying message of unsolicited advice remains that there *must* be a fix for our broken bodies. That there *must* be a better alternative to what we've decided with our doctors is the proper treatment. It assumes we haven't already tried everything we could, and that what works for someone else—your *neighbor's cousin's boss's son*—will work for everyone, even though that isn't how incurable illnesses behave. As I've said many times, this logic assumes that chronically ill folks need to be changed. And that's false.

This isn't anyone's fault, really. Everything we learn about illness tells us that it either goes away or kills us. There's a several-billion-dollar wellness industry banking on the belief that bodies can be healed, slimmed, and fortified with alternative therapies and at-home remedies. Books about celery juice "cures" move millions of copies and sit on bestseller lists for weeks. Bags of rocks that promise to provide "emotional strength" sell for $85. We're *all* suckers, and the system likes it that way—it keeps us hopeful and it keeps us spending money. There's big bread to be made off the promise of a chronic illness cure.

Chronically ill folks themselves aren't immune to shelling out bad advice, either. But we need to understand that chronically ill people fall prey to predatory wellness claims because traditional health-care providers have, in many ways, failed us. They've undermined our suffering, misdiagnosed us, and told us our symptoms are all in our heads. Called us "hysterical." Treated us like drug seekers. The roots of mistrust run deep, and the medical community still has a lot to answer for.

Chronically ill people wish our loved ones would support us in better ways than unsolicited, unhelpful advice. There's a lot they could say that doesn't include advice we never asked for (and have most certainly heard before):

- "I can't imagine how hard it is to go through what you're going through. I'm here for whatever you need."
- "What can I do to help?"
- "What do you need right now?"
- "What you're feeling is valid. Do you want to talk about it?"
- "What's your favorite meal? Could I make it for you?"
- "I hear you."
- "I just wanted you to know that I see how hard you're trying, and I'm here to help as much as I can."

- "Could I watch your kids for an afternoon so you can rest?"
- "I have some free time this weekend. Let me run errands for you."
- "I bought a book about Crohn's disease so I can learn more about what you deal with every day!"
- "I'm so sorry you have to deal with this."
- "I don't know enough to have an opinion."

In the *Los Angeles Times*, Susan Silk and Barry Goldman created a brilliant model for how to not say the wrong thing to people who are suffering. It works like this:

> Draw a circle. This is the center ring. In it, put the name of
> the person at the center of the current trauma. . . . Now draw
> a larger circle around the first one. In that ring put the name
> of the person next closest to the trauma. . . . Repeat the process
> as many times as you need to. In each larger ring put the next
> closest people. . . . Here are the rules. The person in the center
> ring can say anything she wants to anyone, anywhere. She
> can kvetch and complain and whine and moan and curse the
> heavens and say, "Life is unfair" and "Why me?" That's the
> one payoff for being in the center ring. Everyone else can say
> those things too, but only to people in larger rings. When you
> are talking to a person in a ring smaller than yours, someone
> closer to the center of the crisis, the goal is to help . . . if you're
> going to open your mouth, ask yourself if what you are about
> to say is likely to provide comfort and support. If it isn't,
> don't say it. Don't, for example, give advice. People who are
> suffering from trauma don't need advice. They need comfort
> and support.

Secret #2: We want people to stop commenting on what we eat.

On top of unsolicited advice, *everyone* has a different opinion on what chronically ill people should be consuming: low-carb, high-carb, no-carb, specific-carb, low-fat, high-fat, low-FODMAP, keto, Atkins, low-sugar, no-sugar, high-protein, lean-protein, clean, raw, vegan. It's enough to make your head spin. That belief that chronically ill people need to be—*must be*—fixed leads healthy individuals to think that they have some kind of authority to comment on what we eat, our exercise, the medications we take, and how we move through space. Diet culture would have us believe that thinness is the cure to all that ails. But chronic diseases are tricky when it comes to food. For example, "good" foods (side note: Can we talk about how problematic it is that we've given morality to food?) like seeds, nuts, raw fruits and veggies, and whole grains can be difficult for people with gut diseases like IBD to break down and digest, leading to pain and blockages. Crohnies often rely on simple carbohydrates—potatoes, white rice, white bread, and pasta—which are easier on our guts. And people with ostomies have further restrictions to control output and gas. Across the board, almost all of us have dietary restrictions, and through diagnosis and/or trial and error, we know well what we can and cannot eat. Some of us are on medical diets or require feeding tubes. Medications that make us gain or lose weight may influence what we eat, too. We might skip the food at a social gathering or even bring our own. For IBDers, food can be uncertain, confusing, and scary: What will cause pain and what won't? Some folks wind up with secondary eating disorders because food becomes so anxiety-provoking.

Chronically ill people deemed "overweight" or "obese" get the worst of this food shaming. It's often disguised as concern— e.g., "I'm just worried about your health" or "I think you'd feel so much better if you lost some weight." If people like to police chronically ill bodies, then they *love* to police fat, chronically ill bodies. But hiding fatphobia behind "health concerns" is dangerous and destructive, not only for the individuals on the end of the comments but for how fat bodies are treated more broadly. Equating fatness with poor health leads to outcomes like those discussed in Chapter Two—real health problems dismissed, found late, or not at all. (If you want to learn about fatphobia's historically racist roots, read *Fearing the Black Body* by University of California–Irvine's Sabrina Strings.)

Telling individuals what they should or shouldn't eat overlooks the privilege and pleasure of food. Not everyone has access to fresh, whole foods, or when they do, it's unaffordable. Plus, food is more than "good" or "bad." Food makes us feel safe, nostalgic, happy. It connects us to other people. Food is fuel, sure, but it's also a lifeline to culture and ancestry. *And it's delicious!* Chronic illness can make small joys hard to come by. And yes, food is an important part of managing our illnesses. But unless we explicitly ask for your opinion or advice on what to eat, don't offer it—and even when we ask, if you aren't a doctor or registered dietician, don't offer any. Until then, we'll eat in whatever way we choose to, cool?

Secret #3: We wish people would stop asking if and when we're going to have kids.

Because I'm of a certain age and married, I get asked all the time when I'm going to have children ("Clock's ticking!"). And because I'm from the Midwest, where everyone I graduated high school with had a couple of kids by twenty-five, being in my early thirties without a child is *odd*. "When are you gonna have a baby?" is followed up with some form of "But how will your body react to pregnancy?" and "What will your medication do to a fetus?" It's not their business, but I reply with things like "We'll see!" and "Crohn's usually goes into remission during pregnancy—isn't that cool?!" and "It's totally safe!"

Chronically ill people choose to have or not to have children for the same reasons anyone else does. But we have other factors to consider, like the risks of passing on a genetic illness, miscarriages or infertility, needing to stop or change medications, the added strain of pregnancy on the body, and post-birth flare-ups. Some chronically ill people want to have children and physically can't or make a heartbreaking choice not to. Others just don't want to, regardless of illness. All choices are okay! What isn't okay, though, is prying for answers about their choices or making someone feel wrong for whatever they decide.

Secret #4: "Inspirational" isn't exactly a compliment.

Inspiration porn is a term coined by Stella Young, a disability activist who died unexpectedly in 2014. The idea gained traction in disabled and chronically ill communities because it captured something many of us reckon with: We do not exist just so able-bodied people can feel better about themselves. We aren't brave for living our lives. We don't need to overcome obstacles, as the old trope goes, or exist on a pedestal to be worthy human beings.

"Inspirational" isn't a compliment, it's a reduction of humanity. It implies that sick and disabled people need to do extraordinary, good things for the consumption of able-bodied viewers. And more dangerously, it puts the burden of exceptionalism on the disabled or ill individual rather than focusing on the societal, structural, governmental changes that would make life better for sick and disabled people. We all fall for "pull yourself up by your bootstraps" stories (you know the ones: viral videos of a disabled or sick person dancing, working out, graduating from college, getting married, etc.), which make us believe *all* sick or disabled people should be one certain way. But instead of focusing on individual outliers, we should channel our energy into making institutionalized overhauls that will radically improve the lives of all sick and disabled folks: demanding accessibility, equal hiring practices, fair pay, and free health care, toppling ableism, promoting visibility of sick and disabled folks, and protecting and expanding legislation for people with disabilities and long-term illnesses.

Secret #5: Yes, we really do need this much rest.

I used to be more fun. I was never the life of the party, but I could hang with the best of them. I worked long hours without needing rest, and in college I stayed up night after night writing essays and drinking Monster Energy from the dormitory's convenience store. I could be spontaneous or exact, sketching out grand plans for my future. But I can't do those things anymore. It might seem like I'm an entirely different person—and in some ways I am. Chronic illness makes me less free. My world is, as you've now read, smaller. I'm always worried about how my insides will react to whatever I eat, drink, or do. If I make the wrong choice, my body makes me pay. *I am* different now. But in lots of ways, I'm better than I was before I got sick. I relish the moments that I feel okay—even if okay isn't "normal," and "normal" won't ever exist for me again. I'm braver and kinder. I value my relationships and want to nurture the good ones. I invest in my mental health. I know that my time here is limited and that what I do with it matters. As much as I hope for a cure to my illness so that future humans won't have to struggle with it, I wouldn't wish away everything I've learned.

Part of what makes chronically ill people different than we were pre-illness is the simple fact that we require rest. Because of this, we fret that our loved ones think we're lazy—and some of them outright say so, as I've heard time and time again in support groups. In "The Spoon Theory," lupus patient Christine Miserandino writes about sitting in a diner with a friend. She uses spoons to illustrate how chronically ill people weigh our choices and use our energy. Healthy people have an unlimited number of spoons per day, see, but chronically ill people have a limited number; everything we do in a day—shower, cook a meal, work, care for family—takes away spoons until they're gone. We might run out before noon some days and then require rest to replenish. The fatigue that accompanies chronic illness differs from regular tiredness or feeling worn out. It's consuming.

And rest looks different for each chronically ill individual: sleep, bingeing a show, taking a bath, reading a book, spending time alone, turning off cell phones, taking a vacation, reading a book, or doing nothing at all. Some of us require a lot of rest— some are even bedbound due to the weakness and fatigue that comes with chronic illness. Others might not need any more downtime than a healthy person. No two chronically ill people are the same. But across the spectrum, we each wish our loved ones would affirm that productivity does not determine our value.

It's easy, in a society that praises being bigger, faster, and stronger, to think that people who *do* more are *worth* more. We value busyness to such a degree that "busy" has become a personality, an emotion.

"How are you?"

"Busy."

We expect people to have a nine-to-five job and a "side hustle," a thriving family, an impeccably decorated home, and a full social life. They should exercise daily, travel often, and make beautifully plated home-cooked meals. And, most important, they must make it all look effortless for social media. Is it any wonder that we're all burned out?

There's this saying that gets printed on T-shirts and mugs: "You have as many hours in a day as Beyoncé." I love Beyoncé, and she didn't ask for this silly saying to make its way around Pinterest. It's bullshit that regular people are expected to be as productive as a person worth $400 million ($1.4 billion if we're counting Jay-Z). Rich folks have access to help and conveniences that the rest of us don't: around-the-clock childcare, chefs, cleaning services, hairstylists and makeup artists, personal shoppers, drivers, private planes, tutors, house call doctors. Completing a full day is tiring enough for a healthy person, let alone when you're battling chronic illness. Capitalism would have us think otherwise, but human beings are worthy of love, admiration, and respect regardless of how much we produce, give back, expend, or earn. We're expected to rest only when we're run ragged, but why do we need to crash to "earn" rest? Why do we need to prove we've worked hard enough, long enough, to "deserve" it? *What if we took rest as seriously as we did productivity?*

In addition to rest, self-care is an essential thing for chronically ill folks. The writer, activist, and poet Audre Lorde popularized the term *self-care* to remind Black women and femmes that caring for themselves is a radical response to oppression: "Caring for myself is not self-indulgence, it is self-preservation, and that is an act of political warfare." (I can't recommend Lorde's book *The Cancer Journals* highly enough, in which she writes about the overlap of health, civil rights, and gender and sexual justice.) Like so many things for Black women by Black women, self-care was co-opted by consumerism and turned into face masks and bath bombs. But for marginalized bodies, it's more than pampering. It's a purposeful caring of the body and mind. It's treasuring a body in a world that views it as having little worth unless it looks a certain way, behaves a certain way, and reaches a certain level of productivity. Self-care is *anti*-despair.

If true self-care looks like a bubble bath for you, great! But it can also look like going to therapy; ending a toxic relationship; spending time alone (or spending time with loved ones—self-care is about balancing your needs!); crying (seriously—science says it's a healthy release); taking your daily medications; cooking your favorite meal; getting some fresh air; being *purposefully* unproductive; spending time in a space you know is safe; attending a support group meeting; volunteering for a cause you care about; turning off social media; reading a book; or doing something entirely mundane.

Self-care is a necessary part of living well with chronic illness. It means you're aware of what your chronically ill body needs to keep it functioning as best it can—be it certain foods, medication, exercise, or stress reduction. Self-care with chronic illness is doing what you can to extend periods in between flares and hospitalizations: resting, reducing stress, taking medication on time, keeping up with doctors' appointments, and reaching out for support. Lack of rest and care makes chronically ill bodies sicker. And when our bodies feel bad, our brains do, too; when our brains feel bad, so do our bodies. It's a toxic loop.

We deal with the volatility of the very thing that carries us around this world *every single day*. We face never-ending pain and fatigue. Our medications may control some symptoms, but they add others, and treatments stop working. We're concerned about our mental health, but we can't afford to see a therapist as often as we'd like, if at all. We're worried over the future of our bodies and how we're going to afford taking care of them when every other week, [rich, white, mostly male] politicians try new ways to take away our health care. We're stuck in jobs we hate because they provide insurance and how else will we afford the *very expensive* medication and care that keeps us alive? And what if we get fired? We're afraid of being bad parents and partners during flares, when we can't support our families as we so desperately want. Hospitals and doctors' offices are our unchosen second homes, places where we face invasive procedures, loss of autonomy, and huge financial burdens. Sleep doesn't come easy when you must worry about these things constantly. So let us rest. We're exhausted.

Secret #6: We aren't unreliable—our illnesses are.

Because we're tired, we cancel plans. Our loved ones think we're flaky, and that hurts. I've canceled plans a dozen times (okay, more like one hundred). I've bailed last-minute and missed important occasions from birthday parties to opening nights. It seems selfish, I know, and my loved ones deserve more than a last-minute text that says, "I'm not going to make it after all. I'll make it up to you later!" But sometimes I don't want or know how to explain. Chronic illness is unpredictable. On days when I feel decent, I get excited and commit to plans even though I know how I feel is fleeting. Some days I wake up nearly symptomless, but because my disease is fickle, I can feel like dirt by bedtime. Even though I try to control all variables, my body doesn't always obey. Other times, my body obeys but my mind goes wild thinking about all that could go wrong. Then, when I reschedule, I get anxious about having to explain myself, so I cancel again. *The more I cancel, the more I cancel.* I hate being unreliable. I didn't choose this illness, but that doesn't mean my loved ones can't be disappointed when I have to bail last-minute.

When we're able to follow through with plans, chronically ill people put in a lot of effort to look and seem "normal"—whatever that means—because it's what the world demands of us. We work hard to hide our symptoms. Among ourselves, we share recommendations for faux tanning cream and full-coverage concealer to help us appear rested. A woman in my support group even got cosmetic fillers injected under her eyes because she was so fed up with people telling her she looked worn out. We wear oversized clothing so no one comments on weight loss or gain, and bands that flatten and hide ostomies. We choose long sleeves to cover the bruises from infusions and blood tests. We say we already ate so that we won't fret about rushing to the bathroom. We try to keep two selves, a public (read: "healthy") version and a private ("sick") one, separate. The diseases make us tired, but trying to hide them leaves us physically and mentally exhausted.

When the magnificent actor Chadwick Boseman died from colon cancer, a condition he'd kept private for several years, people marveled at how he could have been so active, churning out film after film while sick. The narrative became "He was so strong," which of course he was, but I wish it had been "How can we make the world more accessible?" Sick and disabled people work as hard as Boseman, though perhaps less publicly, every day. The world demands that we keep our conditions secret. We're strong, sure, but we're also adapting to a world that prefers we hide.

The dilemma chronically ill people live with is this: We need to appear healthy enough to move through the world, but we need to be sick enough to receive proper treatment. We want family members, friends, bosses, and colleagues to believe that we're well enough to function, but we also want doctors to listen to us even when our symptoms aren't visible. "But you don't look sick!" or "You're too young to be so sick!" aren't helpful things to say to a chronically ill person. What does "looking sick" mean when millions of people live with invisible illnesses? What age is acceptable to be sick when many chronic autoimmune diseases present before the age of thirty-five and colorectal cancers are striking young people—especially young Black people—more than ever? Healthy folks should reconsider what it means to *look* sick, to *be* sick, and recognize the inherent privilege in deeming whether people fit their preset qualifications.

Secret #7: We just want to be believed.

More than anything, we wish our loved ones believed us. Here's the thing about invisible illness: *It's invisible.* A lot of the time, you can't look at a chronically ill person and see they're sick. Unless you come to the bathroom with me or stick a colonoscopy scope up my behind, you won't see the effects of my disease. Chronically ill people believe one another because we know what it's like to exist with this life-changing *thing*, even as we're each hiding surgical scars, rashes, heating pad erythema, and medical devices beneath our clothes. But healthy folks don't always trust us, and that's crushing. Their mistrust takes differ-ent forms, some more overt than others. But one that comes up repeatedly in my support groups is called *gaslighting*, which is a term used for a manipulation tactic that makes someone question or doubt their own reality. This tactic makes people unsafe and insecure and, in severe forms, can cause them to lose touch with reality. When chronically ill folks feel bad and our loved ones minimize it or think we're making it up, saying, "It can't be that bad," *that's* gaslighting.

Here are some other examples that have come up in my discussions with fellow chronically ill people:

- "Other people have it so much worse."
- "Are you sure it happened that way?"
- "There's no way it's that bad."
- "You act like this for attention."
- "But you don't look sick."
- "Your symptoms are all in your head."
- "Ugh, you cry about everything."
- "I never said that." (Or: "It was a joke!" when it clearly wasn't a joke.)
- "No, you misunderstood what I said." (Followed by changing what they originally said to be different or less offensive.)
- "You're overreacting."

Chronic illness robs us of many things, including our power, our sense of independent agency in the world. We gain it back in little self-sufficient ways. But our loved ones can help us get our power back, too, by supporting us—though before they can do that fully, they must *believe us*. There is strength in being believed. There is so much force in these three words: "I believe you." Before anything else, our loved ones should start there.

CHAPTER 17

Thirty-Eight Experiences of Joy

Before I got sick, I required everything in my life to be big. Big successes, big fights, big feelings. I could always be happier and more successful. My jokes could be funnier. My face prettier. My body thinner. My relationship more passionate. I was never content, always waiting—for me, my job, my life—to be *more*. I anticipated an enchanted moment when life finally felt "right." The present was not a place I focused on; the past I tried hard to bury, and the future I fantasized over to the point of worrying myself sick. See, even though I hoped I'd be some ideal version of myself by then, I was petrified of what the unknown held. I spent many nights awake, my wheels turning until the sun came up, stomach full of knots over things that probably wouldn't happen and certainly couldn't be controlled. I'd peel my eyes from the ceiling and get out of bed to dress for the day wondering, *How many hours has it been since I blinked?*

Often, my anxiety looked like vanity. When I was twenty-two, I ended up at a birthday party in Williamsburg for a friend of a friend of a friend. The birthday girl was dancing under the lights of a multicolor disco ball. She had crinkles around her eyes that stayed behind after a smile and a sharpness to her face from the volume leaving her cheeks. The balloons read 3-0. I couldn't imagine being thirty. How could this woman be gleefully celebrating what seemed to me like a doomsday? On my *twenty-first birthday* I'd crumpled into a pile of Jägermeister-scented sobs over "being old." I spent my twenty-second birthday crying and checking the mirror for new fine lines. Soon after, I started avoiding mirrors entirely. I couldn't be present with other people, not really, because my mind was on the single pore or spot upsetting me that day. It didn't make sense. I read a lot, took gender studies classes, followed body-positive social media accounts, and surrounded myself with brilliant, levelheaded women and femmes whose value I did not assign by their age or how they looked. I knew that the pressure to stay young and mainstream beautiful was created to make us miserable, forever emptying our pockets for creams and injections and implants. I understood the unfairness of men getting rugged and women getting haggard. I'd preach these messages all day, but I couldn't get them to take hold in my internal dialogue. Each birthday, I thought a bit of my worth got chipped away.

When I started therapy in 2013, my psychiatrist enlightened me: Fear of aging is common after the loss of a loved one—for me, Dad—because milestones like birthdays mean we're moving on without them here. We become fixated with freezing time, and sometimes that takes the form of obsessing about growing older. We want to stay in the form our dead loved one knew us in, so they can recognize us in case they come back (there's that magical thinking again). But it was more than that for me. I needed to be *perfect.* That's how, from a young age, I felt in control—regulating how much I ate and never settling for less than an A. As I grew up, that need to control took the form of obsessing over different parts of my body; spending hours getting ready to leave the house, sometimes redoing my hair and makeup and outfits several times before deciding to just stay home; placing self-defining value on work successes like promotions; and abruptly ending relationships at the first hint of conflict. I was so fixated on a level of flawlessness I'd never achieve—and afraid of even the smallest rejections— that it paralyzed me. It hurt me and those around me. And above anything else, it robbed me of joy. Perfectionism is nothing more than a bottomless pit of self-hatred.

Now imagine what an incurable disease that makes you uncontrollably shit yourself does to a person like this, someone so desperately clinging to discipline and order that it makes them unwell. I had two options: Try to maintain an unattainable level of control in a body (and a world, *amirite?*) that kept showing me control doesn't exist; or, laugh at the absurdity of it all and *let go*. After my diagnosis, I attempted the first for a while—that led to blackout panic attacks. The second option didn't come naturally to me, either, so it required committed, ongoing work. Turns out, facing the pain I'd been trying to bury was the very thing that began to mentally heal me. I guess Dad the occasional Buddhist was right after all: There is value in suffering.

At the beginning of my illness, I was so inwardly focused on what I'd lost that I couldn't see the gifts illness had given me. Mom, a determined optimist, taught me to always look for the silver lining. Mine is this: Yeah, my body won't allow for a lot of the ambitious plans I'd had, but it also won't allow for any bullshit—no jobs I hate, no relationships I'm not fulfilled by, no hours crying over wrinkles. Illness made me braver, kinder, and more empathetic, and that gives me *way* more radical power than the faux control I was clutching to for so long. In the most unexpected way, illness *freed* me. It compelled me to begin ther-apy, which kick-started the process of tending to wounds old and new. It made me focus on the present more than the anxiety of the future. And it made me be *in my body* in a way I'd never experienced before. Suddenly, I had to mindfully care for my body and my brain as best I could and understand that beyond that, it's out of my hands. I learned that perfection isn't reason-able or enjoyable, and that there's value in being adaptable, less rigid. And over time, I uncovered joy that could only be revealed once I gave up the ghost. Those joys were often small, quiet—not found in B-I-G moments, like I'd been waiting for—but I noticed them. What makes me feel good? What makes me smile? What makes me feel alive? When am I my truest self? These tiny joys had been there all along, but it took getting sick for me to fully witness them.

The writer Alice Walker said, "'Thank you' is the best prayer that anyone could say. I say that one a lot. 'Thank you' expresses extreme gratitude, humility, understanding." Even on my worst days, I wordlessly say "thank you" to everyone and no one.

Meaning and *joy* and *gratitude* are these big-little words that suggest nothing and everything. They get hashtagged on social media, printed on discount wall art, and thrown around ven-ture capitalists' podcasts. They're aspirational destinations and final ascents—things we're supposed to find, supposed to feel. But when you're chronically ill, these emotions are what you're choosing every time you decide to do another day, to stay here, where life is worth living. Each time you've decided that it's worth it, despite the pain. Meaning and joy and gratitude are hard-fought moments for which we've scratched and crawled and bled—often literally. They are a dedicated practice as vital to our living well as medication and good health care. Happiness is something you *chase*, but joy is something you *choose*.

It isn't always easy, I know. Some days meaning and joy and gratitude are difficult—impossible—to find. Some days everything hurts. Pain sinks its tentacles into the rational parts of my brain and all I can do is wallow in how much it sucks, hoping tomorrow will be worth sticking around for. Because tomorrow, on the other side of pain, comes joy: a sunrise; a neighbor kid's smile, missing his two front teeth; four dogs welcoming me home; texts with Kaetlyn; a walk around the block; home-cooked meals; Greg's laugh; a hot bath; a book I've read before; the mindless bliss of a Netflix binge. *La dolce far niente*, as the Italians call it: the sweetness of doing nothing. Sometimes, it's no more than simply making it through a day. And then another. And another. Yet I hope it gets better and believe that it will, not because it *doesn't* suck right now, but because belief in better days is how I survive.

Chronically ill people are kind, funny, and brave, with a vast knowledge about how to make things—systems, governments, infrastructures—better. We are radical changemakers (just watch the documentary *Crip Camp* for an introduction!). I hope for a cure to all forever sickness, but I also know that a world without chronically ill and disabled people is an unquestionably worse world.

I am one chronically ill person. My experience isn't universal for all sick people, so when I say that joy is possible, why should you believe me? So here, to help me prove this point, I asked members of my community from different places and backgrounds, with different diagnoses, to share what brings them joy despite, and *because of*, forever sickness. You might not take my word alone, but how about thirty-eight more corroborations?

I have a network of women who know what I'm going through and who give me strength daily. **Every seemingly average, pain-free day is a celebration.**
—HANNAH, Illinois, celiac disease and endometriosis

I relish in the things my body can do, both simple and complex, *especially* when I'm having a flare. On days when I feel weak and beat down by my disease, I return to my yoga and am amazed by my body's strength and fluidity. —HANNAH, Kansas, Crohn's disease

I'm more spontaneous than I used to be in taking advantage of opportunities. At the same time, I love quiet evenings at home where I can snuggle up under a blanket, drink a warm beverage, watch TV, and enjoy when life is calm and good.
—JEN, Colorado, common variable immunodeficiency (CVID)

Taking a walk and looking for flowers and plants. My toes in the sand, listening to the waves while the sun sets. My dogs cuddled next to me. Quilting. **Finishing a video game and watching the credits roll.** Getting a new tattoo and looking down at it for the first time. Baking bread. The smell of my husband's skin.
—ACE TILTON, Florida, hypermobile Ehlers-Danlos syndrome (EDS) and endometriosis

I find joy in my pets and my houseplants. **My pets teach me patience and forgiveness on days I'm not feeling well,** and plants constantly teach me that life goes on and with the right amount of care, we can flourish.

—MICHELLE, California, Crohn's disease

As a mom of a three-year-old and a one-year-old, going through nearly flawless pregnancies and bringing two lives into the world gave me a renewed sense of self-love. **Despite my body being riddled with illness, it was still able to create healthy babies.**

—NATALIE, Missouri, Crohn's disease

Books—all of them. Well-written stories. That's all I want. Well, that and some coffee and tea with my pain medication. Maybe a hot bath. A good wine. Running my hands over velvet or a dog's fur. Birds. Clean sheets. **The feel of my beloved's skin under my hands.**

—JACK, New York, osteoarthritis

I'm an oceanographer. Growing up in a landlocked state and struggling with any form of physical activity, studying, thinking about, and **being in the presence of the ocean has always brought me great joy.** Many of my friends and colleagues scuba dive. Illness inhibits my ability to enjoy the ocean in that way, but there are plenty of other ways (always with my emergency inhaler close by!).

—CHARLOTTE, California, asthma

When you never know when the next ER trip is coming or when you'll need another major surgery, **any moment where I can get "holy crap, I have this daunting illness" out of my mind is something I'm happy about.**
—ANDREW, New York, Crohn's disease

Being sick has attuned me to my body and my needs in a very intense way, so I can't force myself to do things that will hurt me. I respect my limits both physical and emotional more than ever. **I know when to push and when to be gentle,** which allows me to enjoy my good days more.

—CORINNE, New York, postural orthostatic tachycardia syndrome (POTS)

Right now, **solid poops bring me joy.** I've had such a hard journey so far, but I recently switched medications and am already seeing positive changes. It feels so good. I definitely cried after that first solid poop—the first in, like, three years. —JULIETTE, Arizona, Crohn's disease

When I'm flaring, I feel like a zombie and have to search for the smallest things to bring me joy. When I'm not flaring, though, I can live like a normal person. It's a strange way that my life has been divided for a long time now. But **even at my sickest, I try to get out of the house as much as I can**. —KAITLIN, Delaware, Crohn's disease

It's confusing and hard to be thankful for my diagnosis, but without it, I may not have found my path in life. I locked on to a dream I've had since I was a kid—becoming a sportswriter—and held on to that to survive the most traumatic points. I was sitting on a gurney when I got my acceptance to the Medill School of Journalism. My mom cried a lot at graduation—happy tears.

—**JUSTIN, New York, ulcerative colitis**

There was a long period of time when I felt no joy at all because of my illness and all the medications. Everything felt so dark. But nowadays my body is giving me a bit of a truce, and **all the tiny little joys are so valuable.** It might sound cliché, but illness puts in perspective all the daily pleasures that didn't matter enough before.

—**MARIAM, Spain, ulcerative colitis**

Crohn's took over my life at the age of 21 and I thought I'd never visit all the fabulous places I'd dreamed about. However, my stoma (who I nicknamed Jabba the Hutt) made me feel so well that I could travel after all. What brings me joy is **traveling around the world.**

—**APRIL, Scotland, Crohn's disease**

When I'm having a good day, **I really enjoy moving my body in ways that feel good,** like taking a long walk, exercising on my own, or going to a group exercise class. It makes me feel as though my body is still strong and is

capable of becoming stronger. I'm also a percussionist and I love practicing with my **all-women percussion group**.
—JULIA, Washington, DC, Crohn's disease

I became a great cook. **There's a mystical power in transforming a collection of ingredients into a cohesive whole.** Living with Crohn's is much the same, I think. —ABIE, New York, Crohn's disease

After I had my first daughter, a flare completely debilitated my life and made me feel like I was failing as a parent. It took two years to get it under control and since then, I've really changed my perspective. Joy is both big and small. It can be **making it downstairs to sit on the couch and enjoy my daughters playing**. I've learned to reset my expectations. —BETH, Virginia, Crohn's disease

It feels weird and even wrong to say this, but fibromyalgia has been a blessing, in some ways. I'm more in tune with my body than I've ever been. **I've stopped trying to force myself to do things that I thought I was "supposed" to do.** —SAMMY, Pennsylvania, fibromyalgia

One of my avenues of joy came from a therapeutic technique I learned to deal with an anxiety attack. When I begin feeling too large for my own skin, I notice the world around me: **actively naming the color of the walls, the**

size of the sky, the little tchotchkes on my desk. That brings me back to my body and the comforts I've gathered around me, and it reminds me how many small pleasures are to be found in simply existing actively in my space, just living in my body.   —**LIZZ, New York, fibromyalgia**

The turning point in my life was when I was finally able to open up to a close friend about my illness. **Being able to speak openly about my issues, both physical and mental,** saved my life. At a time when I could barely look at myself in the mirror, my best friend provided me with unconditional love and support.

—**ISABEL, California, Crohn's disease**

The potential loneliness of Crohn's was one of the things that scared me most and finding positivity every day has been important. **I try to do one activity a day that brings me satisfaction,** just to get fresh air and remember life not tied to a bed.   —**MATTEO, California, Crohn's disease**

I'm amazing and that brings me joy. I tell myself that every day as I wake up knowing I'm at risk for a heart attack, knowing I'll have a spasm in the afternoon or evening. When I go to bed at night with a new ache or pain I'm amazed because through it all, I find a way to live my best life.

—**AKILAH, California, coronary artery spasms, orthostatic hypotension, pre-atrial contractions, and inappropriate sinus tachycardia**

Something as simple as seeing my dog run free and happy along the ocean surf while a neon green ball bounces a few feet from her is contagious enough to feel that joy myself. **In that moment, her happiness is my happiness; her freedom is my freedom.**

—LIA, Oregon, Crohn's disease

I'm 15 years old. I co-founded an organization called Athletes vs. Crohn's & Colitis with NBA player Larry Nance Jr. of the Cleveland Cavaliers. Seeing Larry, who has Crohn's disease too, out there doing what he loves made me realize **there's nothing I can't do.**

—NOAH, New York, Crohn's disease

I'm blessed in so many more ways than I'm not. Despite my illness I'm capable of living my life even if it's harder, slower, or delayed. **Sometimes I'm not able to do certain things and I've come to terms with that.** It's OK. I focus on the quality and joy in the moment when I'm capable.

—JULIETTE, California, complex regional pain syndrome (CRPS)

It's scary to admit when you're not coping or that today is the worst day in a series of terrible days. **But every time I open up, I receive nothing but love and warmth.** To feel safety when you need it most is true joy.

—MOLLY, Ireland, mixed connective tissue disease (MCTD)

I'm currently mentoring a university student who's awaiting surgery to confirm her endometriosis diagnosis. **It helps to share my experience and advice with someone who's experiencing what I did.** —GRACE, South Carolina, endometriosis and adenomyosis

I'm presently on bed rest since a spinal tap led to a cerebrospinal fluid leak. **I'm now limited to my imagination and the friendships I have.** Joy, then, has shown up in the form of connection with others. I feel joy when I can help others muddle through their problems. When I feel seen and heard. When I'm able to laugh on the phone despite not being able to walk.

—JODI, Canada, EDS, celiac disease, and cerebrospinal fluid leak

Dogs bring me joy especially when I'm having a bad pain day—they know when I'm down. And being creative brings me joy. I have slowed down, but I appreciate the capability I still have to create something. Painting, making gnomes, poetry. —TANIA, Canada, lupus

I've made a lot of friends online to talk to and game with. They make me feel less alone even if they're states or countries away. **My friends still invite me to activities even if I can't always go, and it's nice being invited even if it's a 50/50 chance I can't make it.**

—BRIELLE, Ohio, fibromyalgia and multiple sclerosis (MS)

I've found out more about myself because of this illness. I'm actually pretty tough and resilient. **I'm 60, and now I walk 45 minutes a day.** Every time I have an exacerbation of symptoms, I lose ground on my ability to move and have to work my way up again. **It can be Sisyphean at times. But I haven't given up.**

—**DEBORAH, Ohio, chronic obstructive pulmonary disease (COPD)**

Despite my chronic illnesses, I find joy in my son each and every day. He doesn't see the achy joints, limited dexterity, painful extremities, or extreme fatigue. He sees the tickle monster, hide-and-seek master, snuggle pro, and lover of all things books. **I've learned to slow down and see the world through his eyes.**

—**ANNMARIE, New Jersey, undifferentiated connective tissue disease (UCTD), arthritis, and asthma**

My body can almost sense spring on the horizon and when that first warm day arrives, when I get up in the morning and it doesn't take me two hours to walk without pain, when I can step outside with just a light sweater and tell my daughters we can go to the park after school—the smile on their faces brings real joy.

—**GIULIA, England, psoriatic arthritis**

PCOS removed my ability to have children at 15. Male surgeons refused my pleas for a hysterectomy. I owe each

joy I get to experience to [my current doctor]. She fought to allow the hysterectomy I needed after removing stage III cervical cancer. **I'm inspired daily by professionals that help patients with integrity rather than ego.**
—CHARLIE, Washington, polycystic ovarian syndrome (PCOS), asthma, and COPD

EDS requires me to tune into my body's cues in a way that's favorably deepened my relationship with it. And having AFAP has empowered me to take risks that have greatly enriched my life, like applying for artists' residencies, playing the fiddle, and planning more community-involved, trauma-aware art projects.
—HAYDEN, Washington, EDS and attenuated familial adenomatous polyposis (AFAP)

My younger sister and I both have serious chronic illnesses, so we take care of each other. **It's such a comfort to live with someone who just gets it when I'm too tired or sick to do certain things**, and who helps without question and without treating it like a burden.
—JESSICA, Missouri, PCOS, congestive heart failure

Joy is waking up and enjoying coffee and the sunrise. Joy is talking to someone newly diagnosed, knowing my story could change their own disease timeline. Joy is the ability to find happiness in tiny things that you wouldn't

otherwise see. **I think it's hard to find beauty in things unless you have seen some of the darkness.**
—ALICIA, Pennsylvania, Crohn's disease

I am thirty-two years old now. I'm older than that dancing birthday girl, and if I'm lucky, I'll be around to see many more years. Illness and infection brought me close to death more than once, but each time I returned with one devastating thought: *I want to live.* Not just that, I want to *notice* when and how I'm alive. I'm still learning many of the lessons in this book, some of which will take an entire life's work to grasp. What matters to me now is not perfection but practice. I'm proud that I haven't let incurable illness coarsen my heart to the good things this world has to offer—instead, it opened me up to kindness, humor, and connection. It made me focus less on how others think of me—or how I'm impressing them—and instead on how I feel. It made me curious enough to stick around and see what kind of person I turn out to be. And if I cry on my birthday now, it's out of sheer happiness and disbelief that I'm here at all.

When I was a child, moving my body and chanting in patterns of fours, avoiding sixes, and eating food items in even numbers, I also became fixated with 11:11 on the clock. "11:11, make a wish!" as the saying goes, but that cute ritual became an obsession in my OCD brain. If I didn't wish twice a day—a.m. and p.m.—I believed I'd thrown off the balance of the universe and that I'd cause something bad to happen to my family. Catching the clock at 11:12 destroyed me until it came back around again and I could "restore" the balance. My set bedtime was 9:00 p.m., but I couldn't sleep until the wish was made. I was constantly exhausted—that's way too late for a little kid to be awake when they have school the next morning. And the wish was always the same—that was part of the compulsion. It had to be the same every single time, and I could never, ever tell anyone or I would be damned. The world would end and my family would get sucked into the earth (or something like that).

I can tell you the wish now. Twice a day, every day, I thought, "I wish to be happy and healthy." It makes me laugh now, reflecting on what those words must have meant to me as a child, how I defined them within my strict, self-made parameters. Little me would have been horrified to know that that wish didn't save me from sorrow or pain or incurable illness. How many hours did I waste waiting for 11:11, sending those words into the void in hopes they'd serve as some kind of talisman? If I happen to catch that time on the clock now, I feel a rush of nostalgia—such sweet sadness for the weird, tormented girl I was, and for the moments of fear and self-loathing she'd have to endure in the coming years. I close my eyes and make the same wish for her, slightly edited: "I wish to be happy and healthy, whatever that means."

Acknowledgments

Barbara Jones, thank you for believing in my story from the start. Thank you for your diligent work on getting the two parts of this book right, and for your guidance throughout. I'm forever grateful. **Ruby Rose Lee**, thank you for making me seem a lot smarter than I am. You're a gem. **Peter McGuigan**, thank you for finding me, understanding me, and having my back. This book wouldn't exist without you. **Kelly Karczewski**, thank you for being the backbone of this whole process. You rule. **Christopher Sergio**, thank you for creating a book cover that's beyond my dreams. I'm so proud of what you and your team created. **Sujay Kumar**, thank you for the excellent fact-checking and for your years of friendship. You're the best. **Kenn Russell**, thank you for your steady, eagle-eyed guidance in round after round of edits; your work here is invaluable. **Muriel Jorgensen**, thank you for your line-by-line copyedit; I still don't understand "lay" vs. "lie" but I'm thankful you do! **Lisa Kleinholz**, thank you for the extremely thorough index. **Elisa Rivlin**, thank you for your thoughtful legal guidance. **Random House audio team**, thank you for bringing this story to life. **Alan Henry**, thank you for giving me the opportunity in the *New York Times* that turned into this book—but more important, thank you for your friendship. **Katie Baker**, thank you for sticking by me at the *Daily Beast* through sickness and health (mostly sickness). **Samantha Allen** and **Abby Haglage**, thank you for the privilege of reading your work every day we spent together. You made me a better, smarter writer. **Chris Dickey**, thank you for your mentorship. I'll miss you always. **Michael Daly**, I learned more from sitting across from you for two years than I did in journalism school. Thank you. Thank you to **the hundreds of freelance writers** I've worked with as an editor. You've all made me a stronger writer. Reading all of your stories made me a more compassionate person. **Rachel Delphin**, thank you for giving me my first real job and for teaching me that you can be tough *and* kind, even in media. **Doc**, thank you for being my angel on earth. You never gave up on me, and that made me not give up on myself. **Dr. G.** at Columbia, thank you for saving my life. The **doctors and nurses at Weill Cornell**, thank you for doing my first FMT and for sparking my lifelong love of microbiota. **My psychiatrist**, thank you for helping me climb out of the well. **Emergency department doctors and nurses**, the ones whose names I remember and those I don't, thank you for keeping me alive—especially **all of you at Methodist**. Thank you to **my infusion nurses**, especially those at NYU Langone, for your years of care and kindness.

Greggy, my sweet bubbeleh, thank you for loving me unconditionally, protecting me, and making me laugh even on the bad days. This would all mean nothing without you. **Mom**, I know you did the best you could. I love you. Thank you for making space for me to tell my stories, even when they're painful. **Dad**, wherever you are, I love you. Your girls turned out just fine. **Kaetlyn**, my soul mate and best friend, thank you for all of it. **Zoe**, thank you for saving my life in more ways than one. **Ben** and **Em**, thank you for being a light in our family and in this world. **Fievel**, **Dolly**, **Lady**, and **Gixer**, thank you for giving me the family I always dreamed of.

And finally, to every chronically ill person or caregiver who's taken the time to write to me, thank you. You keep me going every day.

Appendix

I. Reporting a Doctor

If the complaint is minimal, you might be able to work it out with the doctor directly, or you can take it up with their employer. If the doctor is employed by a hospital, you can file your complaint through a hospital social worker who acts as a mediator.

If you aren't comfortable bringing the complaint right to the doctor, if you feel unsafe doing so, or if the issue is serious, you should file a complaint with your state's medical board. Serious complaints include sexual misconduct, harassment, substance abuse, racism, homophobia, transphobia, fatphobia, negligence, and incompetence. You can find the contact information for your state's medical board through the Federation of State Medical Boards at **fsmb.org/contact-a-state-medical-board/**. Here's how it works:

- You make the complaint online, by phone, or via mail. Your complaint will be prioritized by how serious it is. The board will determine if the physician's behavior poses an imminent, widespread threat. If it does, they'll begin an investigation under the guidelines of the Medical Practice Act. Medical Practice Acts vary by state, but they all work to protect patients from fraudulent or incompetent physicians.

- When the investigation begins, the complainant and the physician are notified that an investigation is under way. The physician must provide documents relevant to the case.

- When the investigation is complete, the state medical board decides what action to take. Lesser penalties include psychiatric evaluations, ongoing counseling, rehabilitation, probation/supervision, or a meeting with the board. More serious penalties include license suspension or revocation and hefty fines.

- Before a physician's license is revoked, they'll request a formal hearing where they go before the state board. Sometimes this proceeds further to what is essentially a trial, with witnesses and a presentation of evidence. But rather than a jury, the medical board decides the outcome.

- If a doctor is found by the medical board to be in violation of the state's Medical Practice Act, that ruling goes in the doctor's public record along with whatever disciplinary action was taken. You can request this information via your state's medical board, or you can view it online at **docinfo.org**.

II. How to Find a Good Therapist

Finding affordable, quality mental health support does, unfortunately, take some legwork. If you have health insurance, the easiest first step is to call your insurance company and ask a few questions: Do I have mental health coverage? Is there a limit on how many times I can see a mental health professional in a year? Which providers are in my network? If I see an out-of-network provider, what's your reimbursement policy? How much of my deductible has been met thus far?

Under the Mental Health Parity and Addiction Equity Act of 2008, health insurance plans that cover physical health have to cover mental health, too—and they can't charge more for mental health services than physical health services. This law applies to companies with fifty or more employees, Affordable Care Act plans purchased via the marketplace, Medicaid-managed plans, and the Children's Health Insurance Program (CHIP). It *doesn't* apply to small businesses with fewer than fifty employees or Medicare, though Medicare has its own mental health coverage. The law also requires that your reason for seeking mental health services be medically necessary—something insurance companies try to crack down on so they don't have to pay for "unnecessary" or "unreasonable" services. In a March 2019 California District Court ruling, the judge found that health insurance companies "wrote guidelines for [mental health] treatment much more narrowly than common medical standards, covering enough care to stabilize patients while ignoring the effective treatment of members' underlying conditions."

Insurance companies violate parity law if they charge higher costs for mental health services than physical health services; make you call for preapproval for mental health care but not physical health care; deny mental health care as "unnecessary" but don't deny other forms of care; make it excessively difficult to find an in-network mental health provider; and deny coverage for inpatient or outpatient substance use disorder treatment. If you think your insurance plan is in violation of the law, you can write a letter of appeal to the health insurance company; for guidance, you can speak to a Department of Labor benefits adviser (for free) at 866-444-3272.

If you don't have health insurance or if therapy is still too costly even with insurance, there are a few things you can do. First, seek out support groups (or start one yourself, in-person or online!). Support groups can be life-changing for people with chronic illnesses—whether you're dealing with anxiety, depression, PTSD, or not—because they show us that we're not alone. They create social support and connect us with resources we might not be aware of otherwise. But if support groups aren't for you, that's okay! (Besides, you might want to pursue individual therapy whether you like support groups or not.) Therapists will often work on a sliding scale based on your income, or they'll refer you to a more junior staff member who can see you at a lesser cost. But they won't know how much you can afford unless you talk to them about it, so although it can be uncomfortable, you need to be up-front about how much you can spend. If a therapist isn't willing to work with your budget, don't give up. Another therapist will be. If you need help finding new options, enlist a friend or family member. (And when you go to your first appointment, or even your first several appointments, don't be afraid to bring this person with you.) You can even hire someone online via a service like Fiverr to do a day's worth of research for you.

You can find sliding scale therapists in your area by searching on *Psychology Today*'s directory, which lets you add other qualifications to your search, like specialty in chronic illness. If private therapy still isn't affordable, look into your community health centers, Federally Qualified Health Centers (FQHCs), nonprofit therapy collectives, campus-based mental health services, and training programs where therapists-in-training give free or very reduced-cost sessions. You can also look into therapy apps like Talkspace or BetterHelp, which have options starting at a reasonable $40/week, but be aware that users' metadata is shared with third parties like Facebook.[1] Apps may also provide less frequent and/or comprehensive care than you require, depending on your mental health needs.

If you're hesitant to start any form of therapy, *read!* There's no shortage of books about mental health from all angles— memoirs, self-help, psychology texts—that are a low-stakes place to start. Just make sure to do research beforehand so you know that what you're reading is scientifically sound—there's a lot of room for quackery in the arena of mental health, and chronically ill people are already at risk for bad advice.

When you've figured out your mental health coverage and options, it's time to find the right therapist. We're living in a time when therapy is more accessible than ever, but that doesn't mean it's *quality* help. If you try one therapist and they aren't the right fit, don't give up! Think of it like dating: You might have to kiss a few frogs.

What are some things to keep in mind as you—a person

---

1. Molly Osberg and Dhruv Mehrotra, "The Spooky, Loosely Regulated World of Online Therapy," *Jezebel*, last updated February 19, 2020; accessed February 20, 2020. https://jezebel.com/the-spooky-loosely-regulated-world-of-online-therapy-1841791137.

with chronic illness—look for a therapist? A lot of the same stuff from Chapter Two and what makes a good doctor applies here: They respect you, they listen, they ask for consent, they treat their staff well, they communicate in a way you understand. Additionally, a good therapist will have a background and training in treating people with chronic illness—or even better, they'll specialize in therapy for patients with chronic illness. They'll understand the immense mental burden of lifelong illness and be well versed in the mind-body connection. They'll have other patients with chronic illnesses (and might live with chronic illness themselves!) but won't lump their patients together by diagnosis—they'll understand the complexity and uniqueness of each person and each illness. Ask your doctor for a referral to a mental health professional who's well versed in your specific illness. If you're in a support group, ask for recommendations there as well.

A good therapist will be flexible, both in appointment style and approach. For example, they'll work with you via phone or video chat on days when you're not well enough to make it to their office or if commuting is difficult. They'll let you bring an advocate to your appointments. Their office will be accessible for your mobility devices or other medical needs, like a bathroom if you need to empty your ostomy bag. Further, a good therapist will recognize the therapist-patient dynamic as a *partnership*, not a one-sided, prescriptive relationship.

Every therapist has a unique educational and training background and perspective—be it philosophical, analytical, spiritual, etc.—and you should ask them about their approach during your consultation. But here are some common terms you might see as you're searching for a therapist, and what they mean:

Psychiatrist: A psychiatrist is a medical school–trained doctor (MD) who's able to diagnose mental health conditions and prescribe medication.

Psychologist: A psychologist isn't a medical doctor; they're a doctor of philosophy (PhD) or a doctor of psychology (PsyD). Psychologists also diagnose mental health conditions but, in most states, they cannot prescribe medication.

Clinical psychologist: When you see that someone is a clinical psychologist, it means they've trained in a specialized, clinic-based setting to be able to diagnose mental health conditions. Their practice combines scientific knowledge with theory and clinical training.

Psychotherapy: Aka talk therapy. This approach can be practiced by a psychiatrist, psychologist, social worker, or other type of mental health professional.

CBT: Cognitive behavioral therapy is a widely practiced type of talk therapy that tries to identify false and/or negative patterns of thinking, where they come from, and how to redirect them to healthier, more positive thought patterns. CBT is a recommended therapy for everything from anxiety and depression to sleep disorders.

DBT: Dialectical behavior therapy, which gained popularity in the 1980s, is focused on learning skills that help you adapt to and cope with change. DBT uses a lot of the same techniques as CBT and also incorporates mindfulness. This type of therapy is often used in borderline personality disorder and complex PTSD.

EMDR: Eye movement desensitization and reprocessing is a newer, somewhat controversial trauma-focused psychotherapy that uses side-to-side eye movement (or in some practices, ear-to-ear sounds or hand-to-hand vibrations) in an attempt to make traumatic memories less intense.

ACT: Acceptance and commitment therapy differs from CBT in that it doesn't try to eliminate negative thoughts or feelings—instead, it focuses on noticing, accepting, and giving less power to those thoughts and feelings. ACT often incorporates mindfulness strategies.

Motivational interviewing: An approach in talk therapy that uses patient-focused questioning (i.e., "How would you change this if you could?"; "Can you help me to understand more about this?"; "What has happened in the past when you've done [X]?"). The goal of motivational interviewing is to help patients safely uncover fears or insecurities, find out areas of apathy, and move toward positive behavioral changes.

Psychoanalysis: Rooted in the teachings of Freud, psychoanalysis is a therapeutic theory and approach that considers the impact of the unconscious mind (and its interaction with the conscious mind) on mental health.

Psychodynamic therapy: A therapy approach that's based in psychoanalysis (and sometimes used interchangeably), psychodynamic therapy focuses on how psychological foundations—i.e., things learned in childhood—unconsciously affect us into adulthood.

TMS: Transcranial magnetic stimulation uses electromagnetic coils to stimulate nerve cells in the brain in an attempt to alleviate depression. It's less invasive than ECT but is only used when first-line depression treatments haven't been effective.

MSEd: Master of science in education. Often therapists with this qualification have focused their studies on counseling in a community clinic or university/school setting.

MSW: Master's degree in social work.

LCSW: A licensed clinical social worker; requirements vary state by state but almost always require a master's degree in social work and several years of supervised training.

LMHC: A licensed mental health counselor; similar to an LCSW but usually has a master's degree in counseling rather than social work.

NCC: A national certified counselor has a master's degree in counseling and is board certified through the National Board for Certified Counselors, an independent credentialing organization.

III. Mental Health Resources

- NAMI: The National Alliance on Mental Illness is a large grassroots organization that focuses on public education, policy, and support. The NAMI helpline is not an emergency or crisis line—rather, it provides people with mental health conditions and their caregivers information about local resources. It can be reached Monday through Friday from 10:00 a.m. until 6:00 p.m. ET at **800-950-6264** or via email at **info@nami.org**.

- The National Suicide Prevention Hotline, discussed in Chapter Four, is available 24/7 at **800-273-8255** or online via chat at **suicidepreventionlifeline.org/chat/**. You can also text the Crisis Text Line at **741-741**, 24 hours a day, 7 days a week. Keep in mind that this is a crisis hotline and shouldn't be used to replace ongoing mental health care.

- The Trevor Project, which focuses on the well-being of LGBTQ youth, is available 24/7 at **866-488-7386**, via text at **678678**, or via chat at **thetrevorproject.org/get -help-now/**.

- Trans Lifeline: Open 24/7, the Trans Lifeline is a peer-run hotline by trans-identifying people for trans-identifying people. They can be reached in the United States and Canada at **877-330-6366.**
- SAMHSA: The Substance Abuse and Mental Health Services Treatment Facility Locator hotline is open 24/7 at **800-662-4357** and can help you find treatment facilities for substance use disorder.
- Federally Qualified Health Centers: FQHCs provide physical and mental health services on a sliding scale in underserved areas. You can find one in your area at **find ahealthcenter.hrsa.gov/.**
- Therapy for Black Girls: An organization dedicated to mental wellness for Black women and girls, it has a robust therapist search tool on its website at **providers .therapyforblackgirls.com/.**
- Loveland Foundation: Through the organization's therapy fund, Black women and girls can receive financial assistance for mental health care. Find out more at **thelovelandfoundation.org/loveland-therapy-fund.**
- The Boris Lawrence Henson Foundation: Focused on mental health care for the Black community, BLH Foundation provides free virtual therapy support and other community resources at **borislhensonfoundation.org /resource-guide/.**
- National Queer and Trans Therapists of Color Network: A health justice organization that connects QTPoC with mental health practitioners. You can find a Google Map directory on their website at **nqttcn.com/directory.**
- Open Path Psychotherapy Collective: A nonprofit network of mental health professionals that provides therapy

sessions for $30 to $60 for individuals and $30 to $80 for couples and families. Find out more at **openpathcollec tive.org**.

- GoodTherapy: An online portal that lists resources in your area including in-person and telehealth therapists as well as substance abuse treatment centers. Go to **good therapy.org/find-therapist.html**.
- Gestalt Therapy clinics: These are run by grad students training in the Gestalt method, a type of psychotherapy that focuses on personal responsibility in the present, rather than past experience. Hourly cost through these clinics ranges from $40 for individuals to $60 for couples. **Google "Gestalt Clinic Near Me" to get started**.
- Warmlines: These are peer-run telephone services that connect you with someone to talk to when you aren't in crisis but still need help. You can find a warmline in your area **via NAMI**.

IV. Chronic Illness and Anxiety
Symptoms of anxiety include:

- You feel irritable and exhausted.
- You can't control your thoughts or feel like your wheels are constantly spinning.
- You have trouble sleeping or aren't getting quality sleep.
- You can't concentrate or your mind often goes blank.
- You're isolating.
- Your body feels tense and you experience pain or tension in your muscles.
- You bury yourself in distractions, like work, and then feel totally overwhelmed.

- When anxiety takes the form of a panic disorder, you might feel sweaty, shaky, short of breath, like your heart is pounding, and like you're completely out of control. Panic attacks often come with an overwhelming sense of dread or impending death.

- When anxiety takes the form of a phobia—be it fear of social interactions, leaving the house, going to the doctor, or something else—you might worry excessively about that one thing or situation, take (sometimes extreme) steps to avoid the thing or situation, and feel heightened anxiety if you have to face the thing or situation.

Conversely, if you have no personal or family history of anxiety disorders, developed anxiety very suddenly, and you aren't avoiding specific things or places due to anxiety, then your symptoms might instead point at an underlying medical condition.[2] And it could be both anxiety and an underlying condition! It's crucial to be as honest and thorough as possible with your doctor so they can do the proper tests and get to the bottom of your symptoms.

Symptoms of anxiety can overlap with symptoms of chronic illness or side effects of medication. Depression and anxiety often coexist as well. Having a chronic physical illness increases your risk for developing an anxiety disorder, as does a family history of anxiety disorders or other mental illnesses, and a history of childhood or adulthood trauma.

---

2. Jane E. Brody, "When Anxiety or Depression Masks a Medical Problem," *New York Times*, published online June 25, 2017; accessed February 7, 2020, https://www.nytimes.com/2017/06/26/well/live/when-anxiety-or-depression-mask-a-medical-problem.html.

Treatment for anxiety is similar to treatment for depression in that it might include talk therapy and medication. In talk therapy, you'll discuss where your anxiety stems from and learn ways to cope with and manage it.

I've learned several tricks to manage my anxiety but there are two that I keep coming back to. First, I work to change my default thought from "What if this fails?" to "What if this works out?" It seems like a simple shift, but when you've been anticipating the worst your entire life, it doesn't come easily. I try to substitute "What if this works out?" for everything from new medications to job opportunities. My anxiety is always worse in the lead-up to events than the actual events themselves; the anticipation is what destroys me. But "What if this works out?" opens up the possibility of positive change (which can also be scary at first!), and if I play *that* on a loop instead, I feel less fear, more hopefulness.

The second coping strategy I use is to change how I think about what anxiety is. For many years, I thought of it as this uncontrollable thing that came from nowhere—but as I've learned in therapy, my anxiety and subsequent anxiety-driven behaviors did serve a protective purpose through my childhood. But now that I'm an adult and I'm safe, those patterns of thinking and behavior don't serve me any longer. When I fall back into familiar anxiety thought-loops, I take a breath, thank my brain for trying to protect me for so many years, and move on to more constructive thoughts and behaviors. That helps me regain a sense of healthy control.

V. How to Talk About Mental Health Medication
Mental health treatment varies from person to person and therapist to therapist. Often depression treatment, for example, will

combine some kind of psychotherapy, meaning talk therapy, with antidepressant medication. This might require a team of mental health professionals—one whom you see more regularly for talk therapy and one whom oversees your medication—who are in communication with each other about your mental health treatment and progress. There's still major stigma around antidepressant use, which, regrettably, prevents folks from getting the help they need and deserve. (As health psychologist Dr. Caryl Boehnert told me: "You can't get better if you don't seek help.") Chronically ill people often avoid antidepressants because they don't want to add another pill to their already complicated regimens or because they feel differently about treating physical symptoms with medication than mental ones.

It's important for a therapist to know where your views on antidepressants are coming from: cultural background, stigma, friends, past experiences, etc. And beyond that conversation, the decision to go on medication should be a collaborative one between patient and health-care provider. Of course, medications like antidepressants aren't right for everyone. This is a delicate, detailed conversation that must be had between patient and provider(s). Come prepared with a list of questions, including: What are the side effects? If I want to stop taking the medication, will there be a taper or withdrawal period? If this medication doesn't work for me, what are my other options? (One more thing: If this is an emotional topic for you, don't be afraid to bring an advocate to help you navigate the discussion.)

VI. Chronic Illness and Depression
Scientists are still just scratching the surface of how the brain

and the rest of the body communicate with each other and how dysfunction in one affects the rest—but here's some (a small bit!) of what we do know about the mind-body connection when it comes to chronic illness and depression:

- A third of chronically ill people experience depression, and for certain chronic illnesses like multiple sclerosis, that increases to more like 40 percent.[3]
- Depression can worsen the severity of some chronic illness symptoms, and the severity of chronic illness symptoms can increase risk of depression. It's a vicious cycle that can be difficult to decipher and overcome.
- Ninety percent of the body's serotonin is stored in the gut. Researchers used to think that anxiety and depression contributed to chronic gut problems like diarrhea, bloating, and abdominal pain, but newer findings show it could also be the other way around— that gastrointestinal conditions can spark anxiety and depression.[4]
- Anxiety is linked to a higher frequency of symptoms and hospitalizations in people with chronic gut, heart, and respiratory disorders.[5]

3. "Chronic Illness and Depression," Cleveland Clinic, last updated January 2017; accessed February 7, 2020, https://my.clevelandclinic.org/health/articles /9288-chronic-illness-and-depression.

4. "The Brain-Gut Connection," *Johns Hopkins Medicine*; accessed February 7, 2020, https://www.hopkinsmedicine.org/health/wellness-and-prevention /brain-gut-connection.

5. Brody, "When Anxiety or Depression Masks a Medical Problem."

- Some chronic and progressive illnesses, like MS and Parkinson's, cause changes in the brain that further increase the risk of depression.[6]
- People with depression have an increased risk of heart disease, diabetes, stroke, osteoporosis, and Alzheimer's. It isn't entirely clear why, but it could be because people with depression aren't motivated to seek medical care or have less access to good medical care.[7]
- Between 20 and 30 percent of people with PTSD report experiencing some kind of chronic pain, and 17 percent of people who experience migraines or tension headaches have symptoms consistent with PTSD.[8] Among veterans, the best group we have for studying PTSD, those with the disorder are four times more likely to experience chronic headaches than veterans without it.[9]
- Chronic illness changes the way we see ourselves and how we view the world, which can cause anxiety and depression. (Changes in how we see ourselves and the world also present a chance for *positive* growth.)
- Anxiety disorders can trigger physical effects, including diarrhea, chest pain, trouble breathing, nausea, headaches,

---

6. "Chronic Illness and Mental Health," National Institute of Mental Health; accessed February 7, 2020, https://www.nimh.nih.gov/health/publications/chronic-illness-mental-health/index.shtml.

7. Ibid.

8. Jean Kim, "The Connection Between Migraines and Psychological Trauma," *Psychology Today*, last updated June 26, 2017; accessed February 26, 2020, https://www.psychologytoday.com/us/blog/culture-shrink/201706/the-connection-between-migraines-and-psychological-trauma.

9. "Post-Traumatic Headache in Veterans," American Migraine Foundation, last updated May 22, 2013; accessed February 26, 2020, https://americanmigraine foundation.org/resource-library/post-traumatic-headache-veterans.

and dizziness; on the flip side, symptoms of chronic illnesses (like heart disease and IBD) can mimic anxiety (and can become threatening when passed off as such).[10]

- A 2017 issue of the medical publication *Psychiatric Times* listed forty-seven medical illnesses that can first present as anxiety (everything from irregular heartbeat to certain cancers), plus thirty categories of medication that can cause anxiety as a side effect. It's important for healthcare providers—whether they specialize in physical or mental health—to do a thorough patient intake that really digs into personal and family history, and to work closely with the patient's other doctors.

- Folks who have depression and chronic physical illness tend to have more severe symptoms of both illnesses—this is especially true when the illness causes long-term disability and social isolation. Thus, it makes sense that symptoms of depression often lessen as physical symptoms of chronic illness improve—and vice versa.[11]

- A 2019 CDC report said that preventing childhood trauma could, in turn, prevent 1.9 million cases of heart disease and 21 million cases of depression. Childhood trauma also increases the risk of asthma, cancer, and diabetes—as the amount of trauma increases, so does the risk, the report stated.[12]

---

10. Ibid.

11. Ibid.

12. Rhitu Chatterjee, "CDC: Childhood Trauma Is a Public Health Issue and We Can Do More to Prevent It," NPR, last updated November 5, 2019; accessed February 5, 2020, https://www.npr.org/sections/health-shots/2019/11/05/776550377/cdc-childhood-trauma-is-a-public-health-issue-and-we-can-do-more-prevent-it.

- Along those same lines, a small study out of Massachusetts General Hospital, discussed in psychiatrist Bessel van der Kolk's 2014 bestseller *The Body Keeps the Score*, compared the immune systems of women who'd experienced childhood sexual abuse and women who hadn't. The study found that the abuse survivors' immune systems had a hard time distinguishing danger from safety, which could lead to overactivity and chronic autoimmune disease.[13]

VII. Medical PTSD

According to a Columbia University study published in *PLoS ONE*, people who felt acute danger during their medical event, or those who feel little control over their ongoing medical condition, are more likely to experience PTSD. Additionally, medical PTSD can arise from the way you were treated during a medical event, not just from the event itself. If you were treated badly by hospital staff or had your symptoms ignored or disbelieved, that increases the risk of developing medical PTSD.

Some of what we know about illness-induced PTSD comes from adult survivors of childhood cancers. According to research out of the University of Pennsylvania,[14] 20 percent of childhood cancer survivors have ongoing PTSD, the symptoms of which, in some patients, went undetected for years or even

---

13 Bessel van der Kolk, *The Body Keeps the Score: Brain, Mind, and Body in the Healing of Trauma* (New York: Viking, 2014), 128–29.

14. Renee Twombly, "Post-Traumatic Stress Disorder in Childhood Cancer Survivors: How Common Is It?," *Journal of the National Cancer Institute* 93, no. 4 (2001): 262–63, published February 21, 2001.

decades. And this is important: Symptoms of medical PTSD, if left untreated, can grow stronger over time rather than diminishing. As Dr. van der Kolk wrote in *The Body Keeps the Score*, "trauma is not stored as a narrative with an orderly beginning, middle, and end ... memories initially return as ... flashbacks that contain fragments of the experience, isolated images, sounds, and body sensations that initially have no context other than fear and panic."

Symptoms of medical PTSD include:

- Preoccupation or obsession with the medical event(s)
- Trouble sleeping; having nightmares that may or may not relate to the medical event
- Going out of your way to avoid people, things, and situations that remind you of the event (for example: you avoid taking your medication because it makes you think of what happened)
- Hypervigilance—feeling constantly on guard
- Feeling numb or detached from reality
- Feeling guilty, like you could or should have done something to change the event

Medical PTSD becomes dangerous when, in an attempt to forget what happened to them, patients avoid taking necessary medications or seeing their doctors. According to the Columbia study published in *PLoS ONE*, in heart attack patients, illness-related PTSD doubled the risk of dying from a second heart event in one to three years—this could be because patients avoided necessary medications or medical care due to fear and anxiety. The sooner you seek help for medical PTSD, the easier it is to treat and the better the outcome.[15] "You aren't a bad patient if you come away with feelings of anger, rage, or grief," Dr. Boehnert told me. "[In therapy for medical PTSD,] we'll focus heavily on the assurance of safety and bodily integrity. You are safe—what was done to you is over."

VIII. Wrongful Termination

If you think you've been fired because of your illness or disability, you should *quickly* file an EEOC complaint as well as an ADA complaint—there are set filing deadlines, and if you miss those, your complaints won't be considered. You can file the EEOC complaint online at EEOC.gov or in person at an EEOC office. You can also talk to a representative via phone at 800-669-4000 before filing the complaint; they'll walk you through the process and consult on whether your specific situation has standing under the EEOC's legal protections. To file an ADA complaint, go to ADA.gov, where you can also find out what documents and information to include. There's an online form there or you can mail the complaint to:

US Department of Justice
950 Pennsylvania Avenue, NW
Civil Rights Division
Disability Rights Section
Washington, DC 20530

---

15. Sushma Subramanian, "When a Health Crisis Leads to PTSD," *Everyday Health*, last updated June 22, 2012; accessed February 27, 2020, https://www .everydayhealth.com/healthy-living/0622/when-a-health-crisis-leads-to-ptsd .aspx.

What happens if your EEOC complaint moves ahead? First, the employer will be notified that you've filed. Depending on the type of complaint, both parties will be offered mediation, which brings in a third party to help you reach a voluntary settlement.[16] But if mediation is nixed or if the case is egregious, the EEOC will begin an investigation that includes collecting documents, visiting the workplace, and interviewing witnesses. If the employer doesn't cooperate, the EEOC can subpoena them. (Here's something important to know before you decide the right course of action: Mediation takes three months on average; an investigation takes ten.) If the EEOC finds no wrongdoing at the end of the investigation, they'll dismiss the complaint. If they do find wrongdoing, two things can happen: First, the EEOC will offer both parties something called "conciliation," which is basically more mediation. Both sides have to come to an agreement, and a lot of cases are concluded this way. But if conciliation fails, the EEOC can decide whether to sue the employer as a last resort (just 8 percent of EEOC cases proceed to court).

The process is similar for ADA complaints.[17] Confidential mediation with a designated ADA mediator will be recommended to both parties first. An investigation is the next step, led by either an ADA investigator or an attorney. If wrongdoing is discovered, the Department of Justice's Disability Rights

16. "Filing a Formal Complaint," U.S. Equal Opportunity Commission; accessed February 3, 2020, https://www.eeoc.gov/federal/fed_employees/filing _complaint.cfm.

17. "How to File an Americans with Disabilities Act Complaint with the U.S. Department of Justice," United States Department of Justice Civil Rights Division; accessed February 3, 2020, https://www.ada.gov/filing_complaint.htm.

290 | WHAT DOESN'T KILL YOU

Section (DRS) will decide whether to take the case to court. The DRS technically represents the United States, not the complainant, so you'll need to hire your own counsel should your case progress. Again, most ADA cases are resolved in mediation; suing is considered a last resort.

Index

About the Author

Tessa Miller is a Brooklyn-based health and science journalist. Her writing has appeared in the *New York Times*, *New York* magazine, *Self*, *Vice*, and *Medium*, among others. She was a senior editor at *Lifehacker* and the *Daily Beast*. *What Doesn't Kill You* is her first book.